Occupational Therapy:
Toward Health Through Activities

Occupational Therapy: Toward Health Through Activities

Simme Cynkin, M.S., O.T.R.

Consultant in Occupational Therapy,
Department of Rehabilitation Medicine,
The New York Hospital–Cornell Medical Center,
New York City; Consultant, Bureau of Family
Health Services, Commonwealth of Pennsylvania,
Harrisburg, Pennsylvania

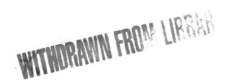
Little, Brown and Company
Boston

To my father — how proud he would have been!

To my mother — the finest "occupational therapist" I know.

To Norman — who fits to perfection my blueprint for a life's partner.

Contents

Preface

Much that you read in the following pages is not new. What is different is the perspective from which the principles of occupational therapy emanate — a perspective based on assumptions and hypotheses about *activities*. Cherished methods of delineating and classifying have been set aside. Occupational therapy does not have to emerge by virtue of an anatomical division, areas of practice, or the diagnostic categories we have inherited from medical practice, or from the traditional division between psychiatry and physical disabilities that virtually makes of us two separate professions.

Instead, occupational therapy here unfolds from a focus on activities — what they are, what makes them therapeutic, and how they can be enlisted to mobilize and realize the potential for function in a dysfunctional individual. A number of case histories highlight this approach. The individuals selected for the case histories are not only representative of the age groups and cultural and socioeconomic groups encountered in our complex society but also have experiences uniquely their own. Their problems result from dysfunction. Our proposed solutions look toward function. Although the cases reflect problems defined by and characteristic of our society and commonly found in practice, the procedures that are advocated, if tried and true, should be just as applicable to the different, the unusual, and the more complex.

A wise man of my acquaintance, Professor Norman Brod, has said: "Theory without practice is futility; practice without theory, ignorance." So what of the theory underlying the procedures? In the theoretical considerations presented here, assumptions for so long implicitly accepted by virtue of our very definition are made manifest and used as a basis for building a case for activities as therapeutic agents. Our claim — and it is a claim, even if it has not very often been stated as such — that our therapeutic agents have the capacity to turn an individual from dysfunction toward function is now open for inspection and substantiation. What are the therapeutic activities that we talk about? What is their meaning and significance to humankind universally and to particular groups? What are their properties and characteristics? How do they produce change? What kinds of change? In what ways?

These questions and others relate to a number of theoretical propositions that can, and indeed should, be subjected to vigorous and scientific enquiry. Your testing and attempts at validation will be the addendum to this book, whether they come in the guise of an article in a learned journal, a dissertation, an independent study, a paper read at a conference, or, best of all, excellent service to the patient/client, who is the reason for our being.

S. C.

Acknowledgments

Growth and development courses are regarded as essentials in almost all occupational therapy curricula. It is therefore not inappropriate to start with acknowledgment to those who, some unknowingly, contributed to my growth and development as an occupational therapist, and so ultimately to this book. For my genes and a rich learning environment, I have to thank my parents and my scholarly grandfather. It was my good fortune to study in another rich learning environment at the University of the Witwatersrand. Two of my teachers, and later colleagues, stand out as intellectual giants who never lost the human touch. Who other than Professor Raymond Dart, anatomist and anthropologist, could close an anatomy laboratory because an unfortunate student had the temerity to cut a nerve in a cadaver, and then instead lecture brilliantly to the class on the origins of the word *skill,* the use of the scalpel, and reverence for the human body? Who but Professor Lewis Hurst could stop the grandest of grand psychiatric rounds because the patient was depressed and anxious, and then meet with her as soon as possible afterward? Both were good friends to the new profession of occupational therapy and understood its potential long before I did. This support was continued by Professor Dart's successor, Phillip Tobias, my fellow student, fellow faculty member, and friend. His lectures on "the brain behind the hands" stand out in the annals of occupational therapy at the University of the Witwatersrand.

America and the University of Pennsylvania were the next stages of development opened up for me through the good offices of Professors Clare Spackman and Helen Willard, whose names are a household word wherever occupational therapy is practiced. They introduced me to a world of never-ending opportunities for exploration and learning — a world that included both leaders and students of occupational therapy and colleagues in my field and my newly entered one of cultural anthropology. Their names would almost fill this book, so all I can say is a collective thank-you for their contributions.

The direct progenitors of this project are Judy Grossman and the occupational therapy faculty of the State University of New York Downstate Medical Center, College of Health-Related Professions, in Brooklyn, New York. It was in the excitement of our discussions on curriculum planning that the conscious impetus was given for a book with activities as its central theme. With the work begun, I have to thank especially Annette Lynch, M.D., and Diane Shapiro, O.T.R., who critiqued, prompted, and cajoled when my resolution faltered. Diane has also been a stalwart support in countless other ways, large and small. She and Joy Cordery, another colleague and friend, made a number of helpful and practical suggestions after they read Part I of the manuscript. Thanks are also due to those colleagues who, despite busy schedules, supplied me with material for the case studies — Sophie Chiotellis and the staff at the Institute for Rehabilitation Medicine, New York City; Deane McGrath of Sargent College of Allied Health Professions, Boston University, Boston (also a thank-you for the activity configuration in Appendix 2); Ruth Levine of the School of Allied Health Professions, Temple University School of Medicine, Philadelphia; staff of the Department of Rehabilitation Medicine, The New York Hospital–Cornell Medical Center; and Elnora Gilfoyle of Denver, Colorado, to whom I am also indebted for a series of stimulating intellectual exchanges. Also thanks to Susan Fine for copy of the activities analysis form (Appendix 1) that we conjured up in our teaching partnership at Columbia University. A special acknowledgment is in order for Willibald Nagler, M.D., Head of the Department of Rehabilitation Medicine, The New York Hospital-Cornell Medical Center, whose interest in this book extended to a gracious offer of prime space in the departmental library at the expense of his own very limited reading time. On the home front, I am grateful for the incredible understanding and forbearance of my helpmeet, Norman Klebanow, who also showed great skill in treating the symptoms of writer's block and writer's nausea.

Finally, a thank-you to those who helped put the book together —
Bill Russell, the artist, who knew what I wanted before I had finished
explaining, rates a special mention, as do Sarah Boardman, Editor,
and Katharine Tsioulcas, Copyediting Supervisor, of Little, Brown.

A final thank-you — to the authors and publishers for permission to
quote from their works.

S. C.

A Note to the Reader before Using the Text

The theoretical premises and the approach to clinical practice that emerge from the text are based on the belief that an individual, by engaging in activities-in-action, is able to attain change in a series of behaviors from those labeled dysfunctional toward those that are deemed functional. In this process of change the occupational therapist is the facilitator. Activities, delineated and analyzed for their therapeutic potential and used in specific and systematic ways, are the agents of change.

It is the intent of this book to provide a theoretical foundation that will give meaning and relevance to activities as an integral part of occupational therapy. Further, this theoretical foundation is designed to serve as a means of assimilating and integrating the numerous and diverse portions of knowledge and skill that enter into the domain of occupational therapy.

It is for this reason that the text is a graduated one, requiring of the reader more specific and special background knowledge in each successive chapter. Chapter 1 can be read and understood by any intelligent lay person; its function as an orientation is obvious. The assignments at the end of Chapter 1 require little more than a perceptive look at oneself and the environment one knows. On the other hand, the following chapter requires some familiarity with the language and thought of the liberal arts and of natural and behavioral sciences. The assignments in Chapter 2 are designed not only to test comprehension of the text but to begin to instill a spirit of scientific curiosity as early as possible.

Progressively, each ensuing chapter, building one upon the other, requires familiarity with increasingly complex and detailed background knowledge — knowledge that comes from subject matter areas prescribed for varying years of study in standard occupational therapy curricula. The assignments begin to incorporate those subject matter areas and their derivative skills with exercises linked to the use of activities as therapeutic agents. In many instances these assignments, accompanied by the appropriate forms appearing in the Appendixes, fulfill the functions of a workbook as well as of text material. To aid the reader, prerequisites that will add to the fullest possible comprehension of the content are listed at the beginning of Chapters 2 through 6. Needless to say, the references and suggested readings are additional aids.

Chapter 7, the last chapter in Part I, is both the summation of what has gone before and the stepping-stone to Part II, which is devoted to clinical application. Since actual persons cannot appear before the reader, their case histories have to suffice. Three of the case histories are detailed, with lengthy descriptive passages intended to capture the characteristic style of living — highlighted by activities — of distinctively different individuals. Also intentional is the great variety in the case histories, illustrative of the fact that an "activities-based" approach is applicable to any individual of any age, of any sociocultural or socioeconomic group with any set of problems affecting "activities health." Following each major case history there are guidelines, questions, and references to relevant portions of the theoretical considerations in Part I to lead the reader, step by step, to the production of a plan for an occupational therapy program with activities as the core.

It will be noted that no ready answers are provided for the questions that are posed throughout the book. Nor are formulas offered that will apply in each and every instance. At the present stage of development in the ideals and ideas of occupational therapy, no simple solutions are possible, or perhaps even desirable. The questions that are posed, the problems that are identified, and a systematic procedure for solving problems that is advocated add up to a good beginning.

Perhaps some of the answers will come from the way the assignments are directed, carried out, discussed, documented, modified, expanded, and improved upon. Who knows what insights may emerge from individual and collective observations and experiences thus engendered? If this book begins to shed light on activities as they relate to occupational therapy, it will have served its purpose. If it demonstrates that problem-solving need not be an esoteric and therefore unattainable skill, if it activates a spirit of exploration that adds to the joy of learning, then it has succeeded beyond measure.

I. Theoretical Considerations

1. Occupational Therapy and Activities — A Natural Bond

"Occupational therapy — that's what you need, my girl. I'll make a pie," Lois Williams told herself. It — it used to work. (When a plane was overdue. When a plane circled a field with landing gear jammed. When — All long ago. She had not made a pie to keep her hands occupied for many, many months. It had not mattered what hands did) . . .

Making a pie has certain advantages as occupational therapy. . . . Making a pie occupies the hands and must be thought about, particularly if one has not made a pie for months. Flour and salt, and cut in the butter — (Mother always used lard, in spite of what everyone said. Mother said there was no substitute for lard when you made a pie) with two knives. Granules the size of small peas. Now water, a little at a time, water sprinkled (Mother always used iced water, but mine is cold enough from the deep well; cold even in August.) Until it can just be handled. As little flour on the board — since I can't find the wax paper and must write "wax paper" on the list when my hands aren't so floury — as little flour on the board as possible, and roll gently and I hope it comes up in one piece and — there! Now the berries and —

It is very engrossing to make a pie. (From scratch, anything else is cheating, really.) There is no worry-room left in the mind. It does not, to be sure, take very long — perhaps not long enough. But while it lasts, there is no occupational therapy better than pie-making.

from *Murder and Blueberry Pie,* by
Frances and Richard Lockridge (1959)

Occupational therapy in a mystery story? Occupational therapy and blueberry pie? Is this an appropriate beginning for a textbook on occupational therapy — a profession constantly striving for a scientific base, which has a world federation of national associations devoted to maintaining the highest possible standards in clinical practice and education?

The answer is a resounding Yes! For occupational therapy deals with the activities of everyday living that are for the most part as ordinary and homespun as blueberry pie. There is little that is dramatic or glamorous for the individual in making a bed, fixing a faucet, threading a loom, taking a shower, washing clothes in a local stream, typing a letter, welding a pipe, piloting an airplane, pounding corn, playing marabaraba (an African counter game, similar to the English Nine Men's Morris and somewhat more elaborate than checkers) on a street corner, wrestling with multiplication tables, cuddling a doll, modeling a designer gown, braiding hair, skipping with a rope, writing notes at a lecture, preparing a meal, bringing in the catch, decorating a ceramic pot, chanting a nursery rhyme, harvesting rice, playing football, or playing the flute — if the activity is woven into the fabric of day-to-day living. Many activities are so routine that they are performed automatically. Others are accompanied by dissatisfaction, boredom, or distaste and may be engaged in reluctantly, if at all. One has only to think of the schoolboy "creeping like snail unwillingly to school." Still other activities generate anticipation and enthusiasm.

All activities that form the pattern of one's life are taken for granted, however, until some form of dysfunction intervenes. There are familiar instances of how a relatively minor injury elicits an awareness of the hidden intricacies of a deceptively simple task. I remember vividly how ridiculous I felt trying to turn the key in my front door lock, briefcase and purse clutched to my bosom as usual, with a metal splint on my newly fractured right middle finger. Previously a daily, automatic procedure accomplished in seconds, the activity became a kind of laborious, lopsided dance, involving trunk, neck, shoulder, and tongue (for concentration) to avoid jarring my extra-long, unyielding, painful finger against the door.

The activity of pie-making is also ostensibly a simple one, especially for our heroine, who has done it all before, although she does have to bring to conscious recall the method and measurements she has not used for some time. For the reader as observer, however, the activity can be analyzed in a number of ways, revealing the complexity of human functioning that is entailed in the process. To be able to measure ingredients, our heroine must have enough intelligence to have learned about weights and measures in the first place and to apply what she has learned in general to this particular instance. She must have good neuromuscular control and coordination to pour and cut to exact specifications. She must also have integrated the concepts of size, weight, pressure, and coldness, and thus be able to transmit her knowledge of the size of a small pea to her hands and eyes as they obediently cut and assess to the required dimensions. The dough reaches a perfect consistency and is accurately shaped, not only because of the coordination and dexterity in her arms and hands but also because the gentle pressure called for is monitored by the messages from her sensitive hand and fingers to her brain, which directs the strength of the muscular response. The control of her movements is dependent also on the stability of her head, neck, and trunk, and, if she is standing, on the stability of her lower limbs as well. The process of pie-making, which she learned by example and by doing, is so well integrated that her mind can release old associations and prompt her to new ones even while she is concentrating on the pie-making.

Beyond objective analysis, the reader may enter into the realms of speculation and interpretation. Why is pie-making so absorbing to the young woman in the story, who is recently widowed, and stalked by fear of an unknown, and possibly imagined, killer? Perhaps its very ordinariness keeps her in touch with reality. Because this is a well-loved and familiar activity, maybe she feels that she is fully in control of her materials, if not her chaotic thoughts, and that she thus has the assurance of an orderly, methodical, and practically foolproof way to reach a predictable result. She associates pie-making with a happy childhood, a comfortable, respected mother, and an appreciative husband. The finished product is symbolic of sustenance, nurture, and love. It promises approval for the maker and enjoyment shared with family and friends. In American society, blueberry pie has a connotation of country freshness, wholesomeness, and a heritage of sound common sense and homely virtue handed down from sturdy, honest forebears – a far cry from menace and death. What are the links between the hands and the mind, touched on by the heroine in her ruminations? For this link appears to be at the heart of the therapeutic nature of activities and will be examined further in later chapters.

Our heroine is obviously intelligent and self-reliant. From her activity, we may deduce that she is able to solve problems. She substitutes with suitable alternatives, as is evident by the use of a floured board instead of unavailable wax paper, and cold well water for the customary iced version, in this instance a creative solution as well. Beset by anguish and fear, she has found at least temporary relief through an activity she has chosen for herself. There are many such individuals who are resourceful and self-sufficient enough to arrange activities programs for themselves as ways of dealing with problems that they have diagnosed with reasonable accuracy — perhaps to allay anxiety, win approval, express pent-up angers, or exercise reluctant muscles and joints. But there comes a time when problems, whatever the cause, become too overwhelming and complex for the individual to cope with them alone. When solutions can offer no more than transient relief, it is time for outside perspectives and expert intervention of different kinds, among which is the help offered by occupational therapy. For these individuals and those not able to define and cope with problems, occupational therapy undertakes remedy by means of activities. And for activities to fulfill their promise as therapeutic media, they must be perceived by the occupational therapist in all their involved ramifications, as the reader has begun to do in analyzing the making of a blueberry pie.

Early occupational therapy was founded on the notion that being engaged in activities promotes mental and physical well-being and that, conversely, absence of activity leads at best to mischief and at worst to deterioration or loss of mental and physical functioning. (Historical surveys and introductory lectures on occupational therapy are replete with quotations from the Bible, philosophers, physicians, and folklore that shore up this view.) And with this notion came a commitment to the use of activities as therapeutic media for individuals suffering from mental and physical dysfunction, a commitment that implicitly assumes that dysfunction is reversible through engagement in activities. At first emphasizing arts and crafts, occupational therapy had of necessity to broaden its scope to include activities of daily living, work-related activities, and avocational pursuits to fulfill its part of the promise of rehabilitation to restore "the handicapped to the fullest physical, mental, social, vocational and economic usefulness of which they are capable" (National Rehabilitation Council, 1942).

Starting out as yet another form of treatment prescribed by the physician, occupational therapy followed medicine in addressing itself to symptoms. Principles of occupational therapy were based on those of medical practice, and activities were tailored to fit this model. It is no wonder then, that an enthusiastic orthopedic resident, delighted with his flash of insight as he watched his patient weaving on a loom adapted by means of pulleys and weights to provide resistance to elbow flexors should exclaim: "Oh, I see, P.T. attached to crafts!" It is also not surprising that a psychiatrist in the psychoanalytical tradition should send his patients to occupational therapy to pass away the time between "real" therapy sessions, or that a physiatrist should see no reason for the occupational therapist to be concerned with a young quadriplegic's lack of motivation when there was a splint to be constructed. What activities mean to the patient in terms of a desired life-style or priorities for "getting better," what can be elicited from an activities history as well as from the routine medical history, and how activities are beneficial were issues touched on by occupational therapy but were not central to the young profession struggling for legitimacy in the medical world.

While occupational therapy looked to the biological sciences, medicine, surgery, and psychiatry for theoretical underpinnings, the study of activities as therapeutic media fell behind. The very nature of activities – overtly mundane and maddeningly elusive to attempts at definition and delineation – did not lend itself easily to neat categories or classification and to the exact or standard procedures expected of a profession in an age devoted to science and technology. Such activity analyses as appeared from time to time tended to be mechanical, labored, and difficult to apply in practice.

For credibility and respectability, occupational therapy has continued to look to the sciences and also to theoreticians in other disciplines who are asking the right kinds of questions. The behavioral sciences have joined the biological sciences. Among the theories that have been most akin to the needs of occupational therapy are those of human development that acknowledge the importance of activities and provide guideposts for administering them in logical progression [26, 27, 28, 31, 36]. During the past two decades an abundance of sophisticated approaches – movement therapy [11], neurodevelopmental therapy [7], sensory integration [3], behavior modification [41], and group process [23, 44, 64] — have been incorporated into occupational therapy practice. Ironically, as emphasis on techniques has increased and as academic knowledge has proliferated to keep pace with bases for rationalizing those techniques, stress on activities has continually diminished. Crucial questions — How do these techniques relate to what we believe about activities? How do they fit in with an activity-oriented base for treatment? Wholly, partially, not at all? — have not been asked. Instead, activities have been squeezed, their intent distorted and deformed, to fit in with current techniques. A perfect example is that of "bilateral sanding" — a modification of a sanding block allegedly reproducing patterns of movement advocated by Brunnstrom [10] in her system of treatment for individuals with hemiplegia, and often identified in clinics as illustrative of the "Brunnstrom approach." This is a disservice both to a fine exponent of a rigorously defined method and to a potentially versatile therapeutic activity. The ultimate outcome is the virtual disavowal of activities as the core of occupational therapy that is already evident in many areas of practice.

Like its fellow disciplines, occupational therapy has developed its own mythology at the same time. To questions like What are you doing that's so different from psychiatric social work when you run a consciousness-raising group? or Why does the patient have to come to occupational therapy as well as physical therapy, since you're both giving straight exercise? the answers are many, and at times quite convincingly presented. A sociological discussion of the desirability of blurring professional roles, an attenuation of the definition of activity to include absolutely everything, including breathing, an arbitrary bisection of the human being into zones of professional domination — all these are arguments summoned to account for our logical fallacies. "The occupational therapist deals with the upper limbs and the physical therapist with the lower" is one myth that has gained widespread credence and support. This concept has resulted in technical excellence in circumscribed areas of physical rehabilitation but has at the same time negated what is essentially the strength of occupational therapy: the integrative function of activities that unite the mind, will, and body in doing.

Over the last 60 years, while occupational therapy has been developing and changing, the practitioner has been changing, too. The occupational therapist has come a long way from the handmaiden, carrying out prescribed treatment routines, toward an independent professional (male or female) expected to screen, evaluate, set goals, design and implement programs, and establish criteria for termination. The patient has also come a long way. That erstwhile passive recipient of help is becoming a client, encouraged to be an active participant (which should have been the case all along in professions that claim to restore an individual to independent or near-independent functioning) in finding ways to reach a life-style that is, as far as possible, individually satisfying and socioculturally acceptable. To enter into a contractual relationship with a client, the occupational therapist has to offer clearly defined program goals, with predictions about the end results of treatment routines. The client, now close to becoming a consumer with the right to pick and choose, has the right to know what occupational therapy specifically and uniquely has to offer. The right to know extends to the community where the individual is expected to function and to the institution that still has to care for those unequipped or unprepared to take their destiny into their own hands.

The uniqueness of occupational therapy rests with activities, in the belief (1) that activities are characteristic of and essential to a human existence; (2) that culturally specific activities patterns can be detected and described by studying the manifest activities, values, and norms of different sociocultural groups; (3) that acceptable or unacceptable idiosyncratic variations can be found by studying the individual activities patterns in those groups; (4) that the individual leads a most satisfying way of life if able to carry out a set of activities approved by the group but also fulfilling personal needs and wants; (5) that such activity patterns can be equated with function; and (6) that activities themselves, systematically selected and combined in patterns tailored to each individual, are means for the development or restoration of function.

Over the years the many advocates of activities as the prime focus of occupational therapy have sought integrative theories for activities, or conceptual schemes for activity analysis (e.g., Diasio [18], Fidler and Fidler [22], Llorens [45], and Mosey [49]). As far back as 1962,

Reilly [57] optimistically offered exciting new ideas based on a theory that linked the mind and hand and gave primacy to activities as agents that can produce change. In that same year the cultural relativity of activities was brought to light at an international conference [70]. Not yet, however, is a pervasive activities "frame of mind" apparent in the educational philosophies, clinical practices, and general attitudes of the profession. The chapters that follow are directed to a closer examination of the nature and meaning of activities, their therapeutic potential, and the ways in which they become occupational therapy.

Assignments to Develop an Awareness of Activities Patterns
1. After you have made a weekly schedule of your activities, total the number of hours you spend per week on:
   a. chores
   b. work (school) and associated activities
   c. leisure activities
   d. social activities
2. Code your activities by color or some other way to clearly indicate those you:
   a. enjoy
   b. dislike
   c. find boring
   d. do automatically
3. List those activities that you:
   a. have chosen
   b. feel are imposed on you by others
   c. feel obliged to do
   d. cannot classify as above
4. Compare your activities pattern with:
   a. someone in your group you think is rather like you
   b. someone in your group you think is very unlike you
   c. someone from a group entirely different from your own
5. Construct a questionnaire that will enable you to obtain sufficient information to identify activities patterns of individuals and groups.

2. Assumptions about Activities

The following are helpful in understanding this chapter and getting the most out of the assignments.

Familiarity with the basic concepts of biology, psychology, cultural anthropology, and sociology, and with theories of motivation, human development, and learning.

Acquaintance with cross-cultural studies of social groups, the expressive arts, and some handicrafts.

If activities are to be at the core of occupational therapy, they must be delineated, classified, and analyzed in terms of their therapeutic potential. But before this can be done, it is necessary to examine a number of assumptions implicit in the proposition that activities can produce change from dysfunctional toward functional behavior. These assumptions relate to the nature of activities, the nature of humankind, and the nature of change.

Assumption 1. Activities of many kinds are characteristic of and define a human existence. This assumption carries with it the implication that a large number and a variety of activities are inherently important to the individual, fulfilling basic human needs and wants. Activities of the human world are first directed to survival, subsistence, and coexistence. Further, they mediate in the multiple and complex interactions of individual and environment and are essential to physical and mental growth and development, acquisition of social skills, and the achievement of steps toward ultimate fulfillment, self-realization, and mastery, whether this ultimate state is called self-actualization [46], competence [69], generativity [20], insight [24], or other desirable end state of a human existence as can be dreamed of in our philosophy.

Acknowledgment of the pervasive importance of activities comes
from a number of respected sources. Piaget's theories [53] point to the
conclusion that all knowledge of the world comes from an individual's
engagement in activities, even those as simple and apparently sponta-
neous as thumb-sucking. To Kluckhohn [40] the personality is "both
the ground and the product of activity — physical, social and mental."

As one watches children ceaselessly busying themselves with activities
— tumbling, wrestling, climbing trees, chattering over miniature teacups,
drawing pictures in the sand, parading in grown-ups' clothes, quarreling
over the rules of a game — it becomes easy to credit the suggestion that
games and play serve as autotelic folk models, or built-in ways for
children to learn about and negotiate an adult world to which they will
soon belong. Play is stressed by Reilly [58] as a means of explorative
learning that leads to a sense of mastery and an ability to act successfully upon one's environment. That the best-loved games of children
appear to be engaged in spontaneously and perhaps intuitively is
remarked on by Holt [35] and Opie and Opie [52], the latter reinforcing this impression with a quotation from Plato, who in discussing
the activities of children describes those games "that children find out
for themselves when they meet." Further indications that games are
activities intrinsic to a human existence come from the studies of
Roberts and colleagues [59] and other anthropologists who have
defined and classified games and have examined their functions both as
exercises in mastery and as expressive models in a variety of cultures.

Exploration of the significance of expressive activities to humankind
has resulted in a great number of works in the fields of philosophy,
anthropology, psychology, and psychiatry. Arnheim [1] speculates
about and suggests an answer to the question of what art means for a
human existence: "If art is a way of dealing with life, in what particular
way does it do so? One of the basic tasks of man, it seems, is to scruti-
nize and to understand the world, to find order and law outside and
within himself." What Arnheim says about painting and sculpture —
"Art is the most powerful reminder that man cannot live by bread
alone" — is equally true of the other arts, music, drama, and dance.
This is also true of crafts, when they are seen in the light shed by
Chattopadhyay, a follower of Mahatma Gandhi, who perceives in the
growth of crafts in a society a sign of "culturation of sensitivity and the

stirring and mellowing of humanism," or with the insights offered by that fine potter/philosopher Mary Richards into pottery as a symbol and vehicle of human expression and communication (see *Centering in Pottery, Poetry, and the Person* [Middletown, Ohio: Wesleyan University Press, 1964]).

There seems to be enough evidence to conclude that activities are indeed characteristic of a state of humanness and that the eyes become keener, the hands surer, the muscles stronger, the endurance greater, the mind sharper, the interpersonal negotiations more skilled, the knowledge more comprehensive, the perceptions finer, and the feelings more orderly through engagement in activities. With this assumption we have established that different kinds of activities have a role to play in the development of a physically sound and well-integrated personality, capable of reacting to, acting upon, and interacting with the environment in the activities of subsistence and coexistence and of attaining a sense of mastery and well-being in the process.

Assumption 2. Activities are socioculturally regulated by a system of values and beliefs and thus are defined by and in turn define acceptable norms of behavior. That activities are socioculturally regulated is evident from ethnographic studies of preliterate or simple groups, e.g., Kluckhohn and Leighton [38, 39] and Lévi-Strauss [42]; from sociological analyses of complex societies and their subcultures, e.g., Blythe [6] and Liebow [43]; and from our own experience and observation. From studies and analyses of this kind it is clear that each culture has a set of beliefs about the order of the universe and the individual's place in it, and a system of values that determines the rewards for and sanctions against specific categories of behavior, including those relating to activities. On the other hand, everyone is familiar with the kind of activities-based description of an individual that reveals the observer's prevailing values and expectations of desirable behavior. To the question: "But why do you think he's peculiar?" the reply may go: "Well, he's strange. Look at the way he dresses. I don't think he's washed his hair in weeks. He's been drifting in and out of all kinds of odd jobs since he quit college. Reads philosophy — for fun! Doesn't go out, even for a beer with us, and doesn't date girls — at twenty-four!" Here we have a set of standard expectations, which in this instance are not being met, for a young adult male coming from the upper middle class. He should be dressing within prescribed bounds, conforming to the rudiments of hygiene, and, after completion of his studies, capitalizing on his brain and social connections to acquire a well-paid and prestigious job. The activity of working has its own set of expected behaviors, which include regularity of attendance, diligence, and emphasis on career advancement. He is expected to pursue leisure-time activities suitable to his age and station, such as sports perhaps (but in no way reading philosophy for fun!), and to live up to group expectations of social behavior, as exemplified by going to parties, dating, and drinking beer.

The permissible range of activity-related behaviors varies from society to society. In many groups, activities are strictly allocated and circumscribed by age, sex, caste, class, or occupation. A man of an isolated tribe in South Africa would be mortally offended if asked to carry a heavy pot of water, an activity that is culturally defined as "women's work"! In India, individuals are rigidly locked into specific occupations determined by caste. Not very long ago, English children of the upper classes had tea in the nursery, while their elders (and presumably betters) dined elegantly and formally some hours later. Our own technologically advanced, complex, pluralistic society, in which there is a relative blurring of prescribed limits, still imposes constraints on individuals, classifying them by socioeconomic status, ethnic background, age group, and sex. The young man mentioned above who does not conform to expectations is a case in point, although he also illustrates the fact that deviations from the norm are tolerated, if not completely accepted.

One example of a group with deviant activities patterns that has recently entered the mainstream of society, even though not universally approved of, is the "hippie" subculture. It has shaken the very foundations of the puritan ethic by questioning the value of routine, regular (and often monotonous and dehumanizing) work as an integral, respectable, and essential activity. Concurrently handicrafts, hitherto occupying a lowly place in a society that offers its highest rewards for activities associated with science and technology, have become elevated as symbols of humankind's return to individuality, creativity, and oneness with the natural world.

We are also in the midst of a conscious rebellion against a series of prescribed activities patterns that for many years were taken as the norm. Sex-allocated roles and their associated activity expectations are being challenged by a vigorous feminist movement, and the resultant changes in attitude are already apparent. A whole revolution is epitomized in the picture (although it relates to a not very dramatic activity) of a husky young man, as liberated from stereotyping as his female counterpart, sitting at the back of a bus unconcernedly working on a piece of needlepoint. This is a far cry from the unfortunate youngster I remember who sewed a pair of sheepskin slippers for his arthritic mother under the bedclothes to avoid jeers from his more "masculine" wardmates.

Whether permissible limits are tightly drawn or stretched to accommodate a number of individual and group variations, there is a point in every society at which deviations from expected norms in activities patterns are deemed unacceptable, labeled in various ways, and dealt with according to the mores of the group. The activities patterns themselves, being readily apparent, in turn define the borders between acceptable and unacceptable.

Assumption 3. Change in activities-related behavior can move in a direction from dysfunctional (unacceptable) to functional (acceptable). Closely associated with this assumption is one other fundamental assumption about the nature of humankind — that the individual can change and indeed desires change. That the individual can change is axiomatic if one believes in the premise that, as Sagan [63] puts it, "In man, not only is adaptive information acquired in the lifetime of a single individual, but is passed on extragenetically through learning, through books, through education. It is this, more than anything else, that has raised man to his present preeminent status on the planet Earth." That the desire for exploration of the environment and the experiencing of novel situations is characteristic of human beings is a possibility made plausible by White [69] and others, e.g., Harlow [30], who have studied the motivation of humans and primates. The ultimate condition toward which desired change is directed is the subject of much debate among theologians, philosophers, psychologists, psycho-

analysts, and other students of humankind. That the individual is by
nature more likely to reach for function, acceptance, and well-being
than to submit to dysfunction, nonacceptance, pain, and discomfort is
an article of faith, acknowledged or not, that governs the very reason
for existence of a number of so-called helping professions. There is no
reason to think that activities-related behavior is exempt from this
article of faith.

*Assumption 4. Change in activities-related behavior from dysfunc-
tional toward functional takes place through motor, cognitive, and
social learning.* Again — to go back to Sagan's statement that ". . . adaptive information . . . is passed on extragenetically through learning . . ."
— it becomes obvious that learning is a process that enables change to
take place when innate adaptive mechanisms fall short or when cultural
adaptation is labeled unacceptable by a particular society. An obvious
example is the individual who has had cardiac failure and who now has
to learn new living habits to accord with an altered physiological state.
Even in the arcane realms of the psyche, learning is considered by many
researchers to be basic to change, in which case the psychotherapist
"functions fundamentally as a teacher — with all the implications that
this involves" [66].

Theories of learning are sometimes convergent, and often they are
contradictory [34]. Some have been applied to explain how motor
learning takes place [14]; others have been selected to serve as the
rationale for systems of psychotherapy [21] that attempt to modify
behavior. In reality, it is difficult to separate motor, cognitive, and
social learning. With activities, for example, learning by doing entails
practicing a series of motor acts, as well as a "thinking through" process, problem-solving, remembering, organizing information, concep-
tualizing, and transferring learned skills to a variety of different situations. When relationships with others are part of the activity process,
social modeling is also involved.

Now that these assumptions have been made explicit and examined
for their implications, it is possible to construct a conceptual framework for the analysis of activities that encompasses their inherent

properties, their socioculturally acquired characteristics, their meaning to individuals, and their potential as instruments of change.

Assignments for Testing Some Assumptions

1. Are activities universal? Do children in all societies play games? Do all cultures have expressive activities? Are there parallels between play and the activities of adulthood in all societies?

    Start trying to answer these questions by observing and interviewing people and groups you are most familiar with, e.g., your family, your classmates (colleagues), and their families. Then contrast that information with information obtained from an unfamiliar group, e.g., a family from another ethnic group, a family from a different socioeconomic class; last, read what anthropologists have to say about groups in other parts of the world. Keep an open mind, and keep looking!

2. Make a list of activities characteristic of your life-style that you think are:
    a. prescribed by your society
    b. deemed undesirable by your society
    c. deemed odd but are tolerated by your society
    d. forbidden by your society

3. Describe any individual that you consider "different" or even bizarre in terms of activities that you think are:
    a. prescribed by your society
    b. deemed undesirable by your society
    c. deemed odd but are tolerated by your society
    d. forbidden by your society

4. Analyze any new activity you have learned recently, trying to determine which aspects of the process entailed:
    a. cognitive learning
    b. motor learning
    c. social learning

3. Classification and Analysis of Activities

For this chapter, familiarity with the language and concepts of social psychology, group structure, group dynamics, and group process would add to the depth of comprehension of the content. Knowledge of anatomy, physiology, and kinesiology is required to complete several of the assignments.

Thus far, the term *activities* has appeared in a context that has given it meaning but not, except by implication, definition. It is possible, however, even at this point to extract and identify a number of distinctive features of activities.

1. They are a series of manifest operations, carried out as part of the procedures of day-to-day living.
2. They involve a process of "doing."
3. They are characteristic of and necessary to a human existence.
4. They are socioculturally regulated.
5. They delineate and differentiate an idiosyncratic style for each individual.
6. They can be learned.

It should be pointed out that *activities,* in the *plural,* has been the term used thus far. This is not accidental. Neither in its generic sense nor when used to indicate a discrete entity does the word *activity* convey the essence of the multiple series of manifest operations permeating the fabric of everyday living in an endless variety of patterns. Yet the notion of an entity called an activity has of necessity been the feature of many schemes for classifying and analyzing activities as potentially therapeutic agents. This is particularly true of analyses that seek to determine the properties and characteristics of a specific activity.

These, once established, lend themselves to adaptation or modification for therapeutic purposes.

Properties and Characteristics of Activities

In its most comprehensive form, a scheme for analyzing activities *in terms of their properties and characteristics* is based on classification by means of clusters of common attributes — often related to procedures, materials, tools, equipment, and end products — and includes an examination of the intrinsic properties, acquired characteristics, and possible variations of a specific activity or group of related activities. Since there is no activity without an actor, the physical and intellectual capacities called for in performing the activity and the actor's responses to the activity become part of its properties and characteristics. An example of this kind of analysis, first conceived for a student assignment, appears as Appendix 1. It follows the pattern of the more informal analysis of pie-making in Chapter 1, encompassing all aspects of physical, emotional, and mental functioning entailed in the processes and procedures of the activity. Included in this particular scheme (Appendix 1) is provision for an examination of the constituents of the activity process: the changing sets, the built-in rhythms and frequencies, the pattern of sequences, the time dimensions, and the interpersonal field. Also posed is a crucial question: how relevant is this activity to the real world?

Sociocultural Delineations of Activities

Activities Categories

In addressing this question of relevancy, other classifications, ones that implicitly acknowledge that activities are socioculturally regulated, have come to the fore. Grouping activities under such headings as *work-related, leisure-time, social, recreational,* and *self-care* reflects a view — based on Western middle-class values and beliefs — of the categories to which activities properly belong and the relative importance attached to each. It soon becomes evident, however, that a number of specific activities fit quite appropriately into more than one category. A perfect illustration is provided by the series of operations involved in eating.

The intake of food is obviously directed to *self-care.* Since a minimal amount of sustenance is necessary for survival, eating in this instance may be further classified as a primary and universal activity. On the other hand, the secondary activities of eating vary from culture to culture. Eating as a *social* activity encompasses a variety of attendant rituals and customs, well in evidence at family and other group celebrations. In many segments of our society, eating out is associated with *leisure-time* pursuits, as a pleasurable end in itself or an accompaniment to outings designed for pleasure. Again in our society, mostly in the executive or professional class, eating is *work-related,* as expense-account dinners and conference breakfasts testify. In addition, in affluent and relatively sophisticated societies, the derivatives of eating ramify into a vast array of associated activities. These range from leisure-time pursuits such as collecting cookbooks or recipes, embroidering tablecloths and napkins, and fashioning table decorations to work-directed activities exemplified by dishwashing, waiting on table, writing a food column for a newspaper, or running a specialty food store or a series of cooking classes.

Activities in a Field of Action

The fact that activities can be related to differently labeled areas of functioning, depending on the setting in which they occur and the rules that govern their operation, has tremendous implications for the perception and use of activities as therapeutic agents. The notion of *activities in a field of action* provides pointers for structuring activities experiences so that they simulate, as nearly as possible, conditions in the real world. The field of action encompasses:

1. The environment in which the specific activity takes place.
2. The rules that govern the conduct of the specific activity. These are *implicit,* that is, ingrained from past experience, automatic, taken for granted, or absorbed from subliminal messages in the surroundings, and *explicit,* that is, with specific directives that are communicated verbally or by other means either before or during the event. In most situations there is a combination of both.

To continue to use eating as an example, the field of action is analyzed for eating as a leisure-time event, in this instance a family picnic,
and as a work-related event, a business lunch. The salient features that
distinguish and differentiate these particular leisure-time and work-
related activities are derived from the environment and the rules, explicit and implicit, and include expectations for appropriate appearance
and conduct, as well as cues from the physical setting (see Fig. 3-1A and
B and Assignment 4-B at the end of this chapter).

	Leisure	*Work*
Environment and Rules	Informal setting and relationships	Formal setting and relationships
	Changing sets	Fixed set
Implicit Rules	Fluid, sponta-neous, and sporadic interactions	Continuous, concentrated inter-action interrupted at discreet intervals for service
Environment	Self-service	Expert, specialized service
Explicit and Implicit Rules	Simple food eaten sporadically during the day, no special sequence	Elaborate food chosen in correct and carefully timed sequence
Explicit and Implicit Rules	Attenuated activity mingled with other activ-ities over a flexible time period	Concentrated activity in a finite time period
Implicit Rules	Open and shared goals: enjoy-ment and relaxation	Covert and competitive goals: satisfactory and profitable business arrangement

Theoretically it should be possible, given a number of situations
successively approximating each other (see Assignment 5 at the end
of this chapter), to make generalizations about the features that separate all leisure activities from those that are classified as work. Similarly, there should be a number of distinctive characteristics for each

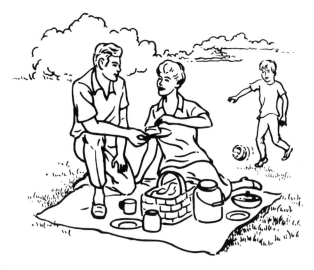

A

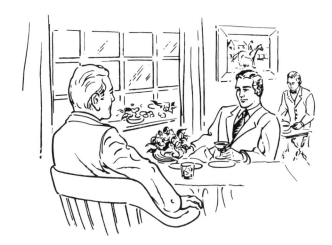

B

Figure 3-1.   A. A family picnic. B. A business lunch.

of the other socioculturally determined categories that distinguish one from the other. The more specific the distinguishing criteria, the more accurate can be the structuring of simulated activities situations for therapeutic purposes.

Time Dimensions
Another basis for classifying activities comes from a time dimension, which reflects a socioculturally determined view of how much time it is good and proper to spend on specific kinds of activities. One of our most famous Founding Fathers wrote: "Dost thou love life? Then do not squander time, for that's the stuff life is made of" (Benjamin Franklin, in *Poor Richard's Almanac*). It is thus obvious, at least for our own society, that time spent is an important way of determining the relative value attached to different kinds of activities, and to activity and nonactivity in general.

An *activities clock* (Fig. 3-2), representing bands of time allocated to specific activities over a designated period, is a useful device for graphically depicting the socioculturally determined patterns of activities for a particular group, and the idiosyncratic variations characteristic of a number of individuals within that group. Cross-cultural comparison is also possible with this kind of diagram. It is tempting to speculate what an activities clock would look like in a less time-conscious society than our own. The assignments at the end of Chapter 1 elicit the kinds of information that serve as a basis for delineating the time bands in such a clock.

That time is a significant dimension underlying the organization of activities in recognizable patterns is evident in writings as diverse as those of Scarry [65] and Szalai [67]. Organization of activities is an essential element in analyzing activities configurations, which, as will be discussed later, are important in understanding the meaning and relevance of activities to the individual.

Activities and Stages of Development
A classification of activities stemming from theories of human development provides yet another dimension of understanding. Activities have

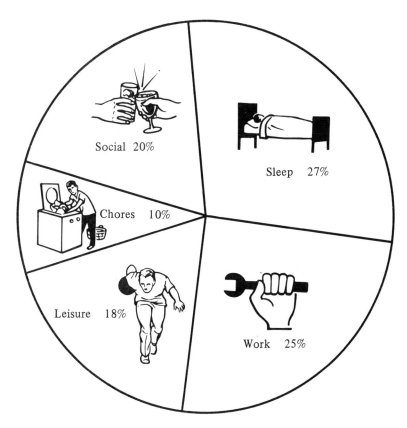

Figure 3-2. Activities clock. This clock shows the relative number of hours per week spent by a 24-year-old construction worker on the indicated categories of activities.

served as recognizable milestones that signal the progressive attainment of critical developmental steps toward physical, mental, social, and emotional maturity [26–28, 36, 37]. Conversely, certain activities have become associated with specific age groups in terms of physical, mental, and emotional readiness for performance [4, 45, 50].

Boundaries that demarcate activities as suitable (or unsuitable) for particular age groups are based not only on knowledge of the state of the organism but also on socioculturally influenced values and beliefs.

One example, fraught with social, legal, and economic complications, is the notion held in societies such as our own that children are not ready to go to work, in the sense of earning a living, until they have reached a predetermined age. Child labor laws attest to the strength of this belief. It is closely tied to another belief — that getting an education is the primary activity of the young. And this leads to a question with important implications for the classification of activities. Is it not appropriate, then, to consider play, preschool, school, and college as analogues of work for the growing and developing individual? This seems to be Reilly's [57] opinion, as exemplified by her advocacy of the occupational model with its play-work continuum, and her recommendation to occupational therapists to study the history and sociology of work.

Function of Classification and Analysis

Each form of classification, and hence approach to analysis, elicits kinds of information about activities that at certain points mesh and at others diverge. Each kind of information adds to a more comprehensive understanding of the therapeutic potential of activities. For instance, analysis of properties and characteristics emphasizes descriptive detail, which allows for comparison of similarities and differences between distinct entities. Classification and indexing of activities according to both distinctive and interchangeable traits ensure that a wide repertoire of choices is available for therapeutic purposes.

On the other hand, socioculturally delineated analyses reflect how activities appear in the real world — what they are, how they are labeled, and what values are attached to particular classes and categories. Those sociocultural classifications already discussed provide guidelines for structuring of activities situations — environments, interpersonal transactions, rules for conduct — that simulate as nearly as possible conditions in the real world. They also provide a convincing rationale for determining the specific activities included in the therapeutic repertoire.

Activities Configurations

No card index of descriptive data, however, is sufficient. Activities in the real world are woven into the fabric of everyday living in distinctive and recognizable patterns that distinguish both a sociocultural (or group) and an idiosyncratic (or individual) activities configuration. These configurations reveal not only the organization of day-by-day activities in specific concentrations of time but also the relationships between different categories of activities, including the relative importance of each, general group expectations and the individual variations permitted and approved, and consistencies and irregularities in patterns.

A tabulation of a representative activities configuration for a group of white-collar worker families in a city illustrates the patterns applicable to a group as a whole (Table 3-1). Individual variations may occur in a number of different ways. Categories of activities that permit a certain latitude in allocation of time may also allow for a choice of specific activities from a wide range of possibilities. Leisure activities are a good example of this category. Work, even though the number of weekly working hours is prescribed by regulation, may have a nocturnal instead of a diurnal pattern, with resulting variations in the times allocated for other categories in the activities configuration. Even when females have jobs, they are likely to spend more time on chores, which include household tasks, than males. This results from group expectations, although variations may occur if sharing is agreed upon by a couple. Children, on the other hand, may or may not be exempt from household chores, depending on age and division of duties within the family, another source of variation. Voluntary assumption of additional hours of work, even when financial considerations are not paramount, also provides a variation that is certain to be approved where the work ethic is sharply entrenched, despite the reduction of time for other prescribed categories of activities.

Sociocultural activities configurations determine the relevance of activities to the world in which the individual is expected to function. Individual activities configurations provide indexes of meaning as well as relevance. If occupational therapy is to assist the individual to function, reality as it relates to activities "has to be studied from the standpoint of individuals and their actions" (*Anthropological Review*, 5, 1976). Thus far, such study has emerged mostly from investigations with somewhat different emphases from those of occupational therapy. Many of them, however, offer information and interpretations directly

Table 3-1. Representative Group Activities Configuration for White-Collar Families (Perceptible Variations in Individual Families)

Monday to Friday			Weekends		
6:30–8	*Chores:*	dressing grooming making bed getting breakfast washing dishes making sandwiches driving children to school	7:30–9	*Chores:*	grooming dressing making bed getting breakfast laundry
8–9	*Work:*	commuting work activities	8:30–1:30	*Chores:*	food shopping house cleaning maintenance and repairs lunch preparation and washing dishes
9–5		lunch break work activities			
5–6		commuting			
6–7	*Chores:*	preparing dinner setting table	1:30–4:30	*Leisure:*	watching sports match gardening reading newspaper watching TV
7–8	*Social:*	family dinner			
8–10	*Leisure:*	reading newspaper watching TV bowling (twice weekly) card game (once weekly) needlework	4:30–6:30	*Chores:*	preparation for dinner party – cooking, grooming and dressing, setting table
			7–12	*Social:*	dinner party
10	Bed		12–1:30	*Chores:*	tidying up clearing away washing dishes
			1:30	Bed	

Variation between Saturday and Sunday – a greater proportion of leisure and social activity on Sunday.

applicable to an activities-based view. Examples are *Human Activity Patterns in the City* [13] , "Navajo Filmmakers" [71] , *The Dogrib Hand Game* [33] , *Group Values Through Children's Drawings* [17] , and "Games in Culture" [60] . Other studies point the way to methods of investigation, at the same time offering valuable data for incorporation into a more directly focused scrutiny of activities patterns. Liebow [43] , Poggie and Gersuny [55] , and Aschenbrenner [2] offer insights into different styles of living, although all are found in the United States.

In occupational therapy a beginning has been made in the field investigation of the activities configurations of a variety of social groups, communities, and subcultures. Nystrom's study [51] of the activities patterns of the aged is a case in point. An activities configuration questionnaire (Appendix 2), although designed as a clinical assessment tool, would serve equally well in obtaining normative data for a number of individuals in different sociocultural groups. Important inclusions in this questionnaire are items intended to elicit the individual's thoughts and feelings about the activities listed as part of the patterns of everyday living. Indeed, the following three questions may hold the key to validation of the assumptions about activities made in Chapter 2.

1. What are the individual's feelings about the activities that characterize everyday living?
2. How much sense of autonomy does the individual have in the selection of activities that characterize everyday living?
3. How did the individual learn these activities?

With the emergence of (1) a working definition of activities and (2) a number of ways of classifying and analyzing activities, each of which yields different kinds of data for highlighting therapeutic potential, we are now a step closer to examining the question of what makes activities therapeutic.

Assignments to Develop Skill in Analyzing Activities

1. Using the scheme outlined in Appendix 1, analyze activities that you have selected as being characteristic of the social group to which you belong. Compare and contrast the properties and characteristics of each activity, listing traits they have in common. Pool your results with members of your class or a group of your colleagues.

2. Using your anatomy and kinesiology notes, analyze one simple process in any activity you selected for 1 (and which you think is particularly characteristic of your own idiosyncratic movement style) in terms of:

   a. starting position

   b. joints involved and types of motion

   c. muscle *groups* involved, and types of muscle action (see Rasch and Burke [56] on group action of muscles)

   d. Built-in rhythms and repetitions

   Note whether activity requires bilateral and symmetrical action or whether dominant side is more active (in which case describe the difference in positioning, joint ranges, and muscle action of each side).

3. Try out an activity in different fields of action. For example, set up a mask-making group with two different background situations.

   a. *Setting 1.* Materials and tools are neatly arranged for each of four individuals in exactly the same way, with a great deal of space between settings (similar to a dinner table setting). Four chairs are neatly drawn up at the table. Step-by-step instructions are given by the leader in a clear, concise manner. Leader is "helpful," constantly hovering, interrupting with advice, very much aware of time limits.

   b. *Setting 2.* Materials and tools are haphazardly heaped in a pile in the middle of a table. Leader lounges at ease in a chair, waving six individuals to the table and telling them to make a mask. Tosses questions back with a "What do you think?" Strolls around the room, not attempting to help participants fetch folding chairs stacked up against the wall. Does not volunteer any conversation with participants. Does not give participants any idea of time allocated for the project. Stops activity abruptly.

If possible, let both groups work within sight of each other. Compare end products and discuss process with participants. Try varying fields of action for other activities. The possibilities are endless.

4. a. Using Appendix 1 as a guide, analyze a representative activity from each of the different activities categories mentioned on page 20. (As you begin to work in the clinic, add a list of possible adaptations or modifications that can be made for specific therapeutic purposes.)

   b. On page 22 the salient features that distinguish and differentiate the leisure-time and work-related aspects of eating are tabulated. Using Figure 3-1A and B as a guide, list the specific environmental characteristics and the explicit and implicit rules from which those features are derived.

5. Compare eating out as a leisure-time activity with eating out as a work-related activity, using for both an elegant restaurant as the setting. What are the characteristics that differentiate and distinguish these leisure-time and work-related activities? In what ways do they resemble or differ from the salient characteristics listed on page 22.

6. Draw up an activities clock for yourself similar to Figure 3-2. Project five years hence and draw up another clock. Ask your colleagues, friends, and family to draw up similar clocks for themselves, and compare them with your own.

7. Ask someone you know well to fill in the activities configuration questionnaire (Appendix 2). Does your perception of this individual coincide with what appears in the completed questionnaire? If not, try to advance reasons why.

4. Activities: Ends and Means

For full comprehension of chapter content, the reader should be familiar with (1) the common manifestations of physical and psychosocial dysfunction, (2) a representative sampling of neurobehavioral and psychosocial theories and systems of therapy, (3) principles of therapeutic exercise, and (4) principles of evaluation.

In addition, access to clinics is required to complete the assignments.

It should be obvious that the assumptions articulated in Chapter 2 point to the notion of the human being as an individual who not only interacts with the environment but also acts upon it. Indeed, Robert White [69] goes so far as to maintain that the kind of behavior that promotes an effective — or, in his terms, competent — interaction with the environment is "directed, selective and persistent, and it continues, not because it serves primary drives . . . but because it satisfies an intrinsic need to deal with the environment." The belief that there is an innate urge toward the achievement of competence and that humankind can literally take its destiny into its own hands is linked with engagement in activities in the dazzling statement made by Mary Reilly [57] : "That Man, through the use of his hands, as they are energized by mind and will, can influence the state of his own health."

Activities and Health
In the context of an emphasis on activities, *health* (or its practical correlate, *function*) is manifested in the ability of the individual to participate in socioculturally delineated and prescribed activities with satisfaction and comfort. Conversely, *ill-health* (or *dysfunction*) is evinced (over and above clinically labeled signs, symptoms, and behaviors) in the inability of the individual to carry out the activities of

everyday living in those patterns designed and approved by the community. Curle [15], while concentrating on interpersonal relations and that particular form of discomfort appearing as acute anxiety, illustrates this point of view very clearly: ". . . neurosis, although related to certain clinical symptoms which may be found in any society, is primarily to be recognized by the breakdown of a man's relationship with his fellows, *and by such an inability to participate, without anxiety, in their common activities that it is impossible for him to enter fully into the life of the community*"* [p. 272].

As beacons of health, activities are therefore the ends to which occupational therapy directs its energies. But, as is evident from previous discussion and particularly from the attention devoted to the analysis of activities for therapeutic potential, activities are also the means to those ends. Justification for this instrumental role of activities comes with a simple statement: there is no better introduction to activities than activities themselves. It is unlikely that some magical leap occurs between attainment of a desired physical or psychological state — such as restoration of muscle strength, normalization of tone, appropriate expression of feelings, or the ability to work cooperatively with others — and the integration of these newly acquired capacities into performance of activities in ways that are personally satisfying and socioculturally acceptable. This realization came to me many years ago after a conversation with an orthopedic surgeon who was working with a well-known football team. He was puzzled by a seemingly missing component in an excellent program designed to restore physical function after meniscectomy. For, even with quadriceps strengthened to the maximum and a smooth and effortless gait, these healthy young men would come off the field time and again after their first practice session and complain: "Doc, I forgot how to run!"

Reilly's hypothesis provides an admirable starting point in examining how (and maybe why) activities produce change leading from dysfunction toward function — by engaging the body, mind, and will in doing. The term *body* is used advisedly, for it is important to remember that the hands — those finely tuned instruments for the reception of stimuli,

*Emphasis by present author.

for expression and communication, for skilled performance — are linked structurally and functionally with the upper limbs, which are in turn linked with the neck, head, and trunk, which are linked with the lower limbs. And all are exquisitely coordinated and synchronized by the brain; which is also the seat of the mind and will. Reilly [57] summarizes the links between the brain and hands as follows: "The occupational therapy hypothesis makes the assumption that the mind and will of man are occupied through central nervous system action and that man can and should be involved consciously in problem solving and creative activity."

In the ideal conception of health, optimal function evokes a picture of intact physical structures and physiological mechanisms, well-developed cognitive and social skills, and emotional stability, all nicely balanced in a well-integrated ego. Yet there are countless examples of individuals who, even with severe and permanent handicaps, are healthy in an activities sense, for, as Curle [15] so aptly says: ". . . often the most effective and vigorous human action is of a compensatory or substitute nature" [p. 271] . Underlying this capacity to engage effectively in activities despite disability is the human will — the will to change and the will to learn.

The Will to Learn

At this point it is appropriate to recall the two assumptions in Chapter 2 that postulate that humankind has a tendency to desire change in a direction from dysfunction toward function and that such change takes place through learning. For activities to become therapeutic or instrumental in producing this kind of change it therefore becomes necessary to arouse and harness the individual's *will to learn,* a concept analyzed and developed by Bruner [9] in ways that are of great significance to occupational therapy. In invoking the will to learn, Bruner, while not altogether negating the usefulness of extrinsic rewards, dwells on the intrinsic motives for learning. The idea of such motives for learning tacitly underlies most occupational therapy practice. In effect, occupational therapy assumes that in the doing comes the reward, either in the process itself or in the attainment of a successful end result. According to Bruner, there are several intrinsic motives for learning: curiosity, the desire to achieve competence (vide White [69]), aspiration to emulate a model, and the desire for what he calls reciprocity, a "deep human need to respond to others and operate jointly with them towards an objective."

Rules for Learning of Activities

Out of Bruner's discussions come a number of procedural indicators that are of such importance to occupational therapy that they are summarized below almost verbatim:

1. Activity needs a sustained sequence, a habitual routine, so that attention can be held by shutting off irrelevant impressions. In this way "the energizing rule of uncertainty" that distinguishes curiosity can be harnessed by one's own efforts to control it.
2. To achieve the sense of accomplishment, or competence, requires a task that has some beginning and some terminus. Tasks that are interrupted are more likely to be returned to and finished; and thus they are more likely to be remembered; those that have been completed without interruption are less likely to be remembered. But the drive to completion does not hold true if the tasks are "silly" in the sense of being meaningless, arbitrary, and without visible means for checking progress.
3. An activity (provided that it is "approved" — that is, appropriate for a given age group, class, or sex) must have some meaningful structure to it if it requires skill that is a little beyond that now possessed by the person, that is, if it necessitates learning by the exercise of effort.
4. The "teacher" must be a day-to-day working model with whom to *interact,* not a model to *imitate.* Competence models control a rare resource — some desired competence — that is attainable by interaction.
5. Situations have a demand value that requires not so much conforming as fitting one's efforts into an enterprise. A child in a baseball game "behaves baseball"; in a drugstore the same child "behaves drugstore." It is in the give-and-take situation of group activities that reciprocity is found.

From these indicators it is possible to extract a series of rules that govern the learning of skills and their attendant behaviors (activities-related) through a process of intervention by one individual (the occupational therapist) on behalf of another (the patient/client).

Rules for Management of Dysfunction

Additional rules are applicable when the patient/client has specific kinds of physical and psychosocial dysfunction. The principles of orthodox therapeutic exercise, for instance, take into consideration the fact that damaged tissues can tolerate only a certain amount of stress (hence graduated resistance and regulated frequency of effort); that the law of gravity operates on humans as well as all other objects (hence emphasis on correct positioning to prevent deformity and a system for evaluating muscle strength based on positioning); and that fatigue occurs when muscles are overused (hence duration of treatment in graduated stages).

In other cases, guidelines for procedure derive from theoretical propositions about the nature of the human individual, the stages of development that lead to this kind of individual, the criteria that differentiate a functional from a dysfunctional individual, and in many instances the measures that can be taken to help the individual turn from dysfunction toward function. Numerous psychosocial theories are a case in point, exemplified in psychoanalysis by such exponents as Freud [24, 25] and Erikson [19], in the client-centered approach of Rogers [60] and his followers, in the behaviorist school [41], and in countless offshoots and combinations of these approaches [5, 29, 64, 66].

In the neurobehavioral approaches to the management of dysfunction of Ayres [3], Brunnstrom [11], Bobath and Bobath [7], Rood [61], and others, primary emphasis is given to the development and functioning of the nervous system, the effects of nervous system dysfunction on behavior, and proposals about ways to influence the nervous system so that dysfunction can turn in the direction of function. Whatever the approach, however, and whatever the kind of dysfunction to which the approach addresses itself, each offers gradual change from dysfunction toward function, provided that the methods advocated are applied in a systematic and sustained fashion.

In occupational therapy it is necessary to reconcile and integrate the rules for the learning of activities with those for dealing with physical and psychosocial dysfunction. In adopting a procedure, or, what is more likely, a combination of procedures that provides a systematic approach to the management of dysfunction, the occupational therapist has to ask those crucial questions already touched on in Chapter 1 (page 8). How do these procedures relate to the rules for the learning of activities? How do they fit in with an activities-centered base? Wholly, partially, not at all? In what ways? It is in the search for answers to these questions that the procedures, dovetailed with activities, assume their true perspective, not as ends in themselves, but as means to the ends of occupational therapy.

It is now time to address the question of what makes activities therapeutic. Activities are therapeutic when they enable change to take place in a direction from dysfunctional to functional. But activities will enable this kind of change to take place only if:

1. They have meaning and relevance to the individual who is to change.
2. They are systematically organized and administered according to principles that (a) fulfill the conditions that arouse and sustain the will to learn, and (b) derive from a methodical treatment approach based on a theoretical rationale or empirical evidence.

Meaning and Relevance of Activities

Both *meaning* and *relevance* are emotionally charged terms colored by bias and misapprehension. As such, they are likely to be glossed over in discussions centering on the question of what makes activities therapeutic. Generally, and somewhat loosely, activities have been considered to have meaning to an individual if they are familiar to the individual, arouse positive associations, and tend to elicit approval from others who are respected and admired. Inferences such as these about the meaning of specific activities to an individual are usually made from items of information about the individual's background and general style of living. These include age, educational history, socioeconomic status, family history and work history, and a listing of hobbies and interests. Without necessarily going into a philosophical discussion of meaning or making an extensive analysis of the underlying psycho-dynamics or symbolism, it is possible to probe in greater depth the meaning of activities to an individual.

An exploratory tool that takes many forms is the *activities history* — the story of the individual's activities life. One form consists of an *activities inventory,* which produces a chronological listing of specific activities that have helped to form the patterns of the individual's everyday life from the earliest remembrance to the present. Another, the *object history,* uncovers feelings and associations about the significant objects, human and nonhuman, that have been connected with activities. These objects may be toys, games, tokens, collections, books, clothes, pets; parents, teachers, friends, or mates.

Several different aspects of the activities history are discussed and the instrument used in each case is described by Matsutsuyu [47] , Moore-head [48] , and Takata [68] . Interviews and questionnaires elicit information about the activities voluntarily chosen; those required by others; those avoided, sought out, ignored, or admired in others; characteristic styles of dealing with choices, problems, failures, and successes. The newly discovered awarenesses aroused in the process of giving the history can be tapped to encourage the individual to take both a retrospective and a prospective view, to weigh, to speculate, to plan ahead, examining courses of future action, and listing preferences in order of priority. The activities configuration form in Appendix 2 is designed to probe the meaning of activities to the individual in this way.

Other than the deeply personal vicissitudes that endow activities with meaning for the individual, there has to be a yardstick for assessing relevance — the relationship of activities to the real world to which the individual has to return and belong. Relevance as perceived by the helping professional may only partially coincide with relevance as perceived by individuals in groups differentiated by age, ethnic background, or socioeconomic status. In a complex society such as ours, relevance becomes even more relative for those belonging to groups that do not wish (e.g., the hippies) or have no way (e.g., the poor) to enter the mainstream of society. It is here that the sociocultural activities configuration mentioned in Chapter 3 (pages 26–30) can be helpful in revealing the activities patterns — and the values attached to the activities —

of the group to which the individual belongs, and also the extent of individual deviation from the norm that is tolerated by the group.

The following vignette serves to stress how important it is to be attuned to the individual's activities background, not only in its outward trappings but in the nuances that give it significance. For illustrative purposes an extreme case of cultural variation has been chosen, although the sensitivity and awareness required of the occupational therapist are not less even when the differences are not so obvious.

He is wheeled into the occupational therapy department, a thin pathetic figure, slumped to one side, head lolling, a trickle of saliva at the corner of his drooping mouth, right arm hanging flaccidly. His eyes are dull, his furrowed skin ashy gray.

Newly recruited from his tribal home to work in the mines near the big city, he has awakened, after weeks of unconsciousness caused by a blow on the head, to a terrifyingly unfamiliar world. All attempts to communicate with him have failed. He seems to be quite unaware of the returning function in his right lower limb and trunk, so physical therapy has had to continue solely with its program of passive exercise. There is no objective way to determine whether he is aphasic or has deteriorated mentally, although he is regarded as a half-wit, probably bewitched, by his compatriots.

In the occupational therapy department his bewilderment is compounded by the strange apparatus and yet another white-coated "nurse" who gesticulates incomprehensibly and moves him as if he were a stuffed doll. The attendant, attempting to translate, shrugs his shoulders and rolls his eyes upward to indicate that the case is hopeless.

Outside on the lawn in the bright sunshine a group of white-coated attendants and outpatients waiting their turn in the clinic are clustered around two players intent on outmaneuvering each other on a makeshift board (a discarded box lid) with "men" represented by soda bottle caps beaten flat. Loud chatter and frequent outbursts of laughter indicate that the bystanders are an essential element in this game of marabaraba – an African pastime so popular that it is played with improvised equipment in any available city spot during any break in the day's work.

One of the bystanders is an attendant, one foot encased in a walking cast, who is hopping about excitedly. The light dawns on the occupational therapist – a tribal game . . . a handicapped opponent . . . lower limb motion . . . adapted checkers . . . improvisation an African way of life . . . time enough to enlist the ready-made crowd of spectators. Checkers adapted for lower limb exercises are available at the large general hospital across the road. A messenger, hastily dispatched, returns with four-inch-square wooden blocks, to which wire hoops are affixed for slipping over the ankle. A greatly enlarged board is marked out in chalk on the paved path outside the occupational therapy department. The patient is transferred from his clumsy wheelchair to an office chair with armrests and smoothly gliding castors. The puzzled attendant with the cast is coaxed into a similar chair. The opponents are wheeled into place, facing each other. Slowly the attendant slips the wire hoop, adjusted to accommodate to the size of the cast, over his foot. He flexes his hip, knee extended, lifting the block in the process; he pauses, surveys the board, extends his hip, and drops his "man" onto the appointed place. The bystanders, their curiosity aroused, crowd around, clicking tongues and shaking heads in pity and disbelief. Now it is the patient's turn. The block is slipped over his right ankle. With gentle pressure over the patient's hip joint the therapist draws the chair and extended leg back and forth alongside the board, then waits for a sign. The patient's eyes brighten, his head straightens, he focuses on the board, moves his hip independently, hovers over the board, frowns in concentration, and then, with visible effort, drops the block onto the exact spot he has selected. A roar of approval from the bystanders brings a crooked smile, a gleam in his eyes, a renewed frown of concentration, and the game is on. . . .

In this instance it happened to be an inspired guess on the part of the occupational therapist that made the connection between a form of activity observed half-consciously each day and its meaning and relevance to an individual with whom no form of communication seemed possible. Not only was the game familiar to the patient and associated with pleasure, but the concomitant, vociferous involvement of the bystanders contributed to the arousal of his interest. The support from a group of his peers was strong enough, in combination with the explicit rules of the game and its predictable outcome, to make tolerable the novelty of the adaptations and the unfamiliar setting.

It is appropriate here to emphasize once again the importance of the field of action, which, if structured to fit situations in the real world as closely as possible, gives the activity its relevance. In this game, although it was adapted to fit the requirements of a very special situation, the essential components of the field of action remained the same. The explicit and implicit rules were unchanged; the essential persons, opponents and spectators (the latter adding their seal of approval), were there, and the therapist, who remained a shadowy figure once the game had been set in motion, did not materially affect the progress of the activity. The objects (the equipment used for the game), though substantially modified, retained enough of their original characteristics to ensure that they were not distorted or unusable, while the introduction of the chairs made sense in view of the patient's disability. And the setting contained enough familiar elements to ensure that it was recognizable, and therefore acceptable.

Arousing and Sustaining the Will to Learn

Besides having meaning and relevance to the individual, this activity, by virtue of its inherent characteristics as a game, had a known beginning and end and built-in ways of assessing progress. It also demanded of the individual the exertion of effort. The attendant with the cast served as a competence model, interacting with the patient to demonstrate that the game could be played effectively even with physical limitations. He also risked participation in a strange version of a known activity, which could just as easily have called forth ridicule as support from peers. The patient rose to the demands of the give-and-take situation, "behaving marabaraba" as typically as his fellow participants.

The conditions for arousing the will to learn were inherent in the situation and the processes of the game. To sustain the will to learn would require a systematic and continued program, in which the frequency of repetitions, variation of situation, and incorporation of other activities would have had to be considered.

How many times can an activity be repeated without boredom setting in? How often? Should the game be cut off at the height of suspense for completion the next day? Or will finishing the game spur the individual on to further challenges? How can the newly aroused interest be harnessed for participation in other activities that may not be as exciting, but which are important if the patient is to return to his community? What treatment approaches will lend themselves to managing the patient's sensory-integrative and other neurological problems? How can they be combined with an emphasis on activities?

Organization and Administration of Activities

All these, and other, questions have to be asked if activities are to be organized and administered in a systematic fashion. Many of the answers come from an evaluation of the individual's level of functioning and from an activities history. In the case of the man with the head injury, the activity situation served not only as a bridge to communication but also as an introductory evaluation of his physical and mental status, giving pointers to further procedures. That he could understand directives, conveyed mainly by gesture and demonstration, was evident. That he could make connections between successive events, plan abstractly, initiate action, and make decisions was also apparent from the nature of his play. At least part of his memory was intact, since he was able to recall the rules of the game and the expected behaviors associated with them. He was also able to accommodate to the novel aspects of a previously known situation. Notwithstanding an abundance of stimuli in his immediate environment, he was able to screen out those that were irrelevant as he planned and executed his moves. Nor, despite a head injury, did he seem disturbed by the boisterous noise emanating from the spectators. Physically, he had enough voluntary control of his right lower limb to initiate movement and was able to move partially out of the synergic patterns in which the limb was held. Similarly, he could maintain his corrected head and neck position even while his attention was diverted to the game.

In this first session with the patient, the occupational therapist acted mainly as a facilitator, structuring an activities situation designed to arouse and capture the patient's interest while at the same time adhering to a number of rules required to deal with his physical condition. These included attention to correct positioning, sensory input to facilitate hip movement, and use of devices to compensate for absent motion.

With the opening of channels of communication, further evaluation of the patient's level of physical and psychosocial functioning was made possible. And once his needs were established, his newly captured will to learn could be fostered in a methodical progression of activities situations designed to help him reach a state of activities health.

The effective organization and administration of activities in a therapeutic program depend on integration of carefully selected media by systematic methods and with the aid of appropriate tools and techniques. These components will be examined and discussed in the following chapters.

Assignments to Develop an Awareness of What Makes Activities Therapeutic

1. Take as comprehensive an activities history as possible (using the kinds of instruments mentioned in the text, others that you are familiar with, and interviews and questionnaires of your own) from:
   a. a member of your family
   b. a friend or colleague
   c. an individual from a background different from your own
   d. patient/clients in different settings
   (See Appendix 3 for a checklist of suggested activities categories to look for.)
2. In the clinic, analyze the field of action for different activities situations. In each case:
   a. Describe setting, people, and objects, and try to extract the implicit as well as explicit rules.
   b. Determine how relevant the activity is, and how much meaning it has to the individual for whom the activity has been structured. List the criteria you have used to make this determination.
3. Check each activity to see if:
   a. it has a known beginning and end
   b. it is approved (i.e., appropriate to a given age group, sex, class, and so on)
   c. has a sustained sequence
   d. demands a degree of effort from the patient/client
   e. has a visible means of checking progress
   Get your information from the therapist, the patient/client, and your own observations. Make a note of instances where your sources of

information do not coincide and speculate about possible reasons for the differences.

3. For the patient with the head injury discussed in this chapter, write a treatment plan that fulfills the conditions for a therapeutic activities program, including:

a. activities that have meaning and relevance

b. a systematic treatment approach based on a theoretical rationale

c. a weekly program schedule

4. Analyze, under the headings outlined on the work sheet (Appendix 4), a number of theoretical approaches to physical and psychosocial function/dysfunction that are familiar to you. Read the chapter "Integration of Information" in *Development of Sensory Integrative Theory and Practice* by A. J. Ayres [3] for a model of how to analyze theoretical concepts for their clinical implications.

5. Methods and Media

For this chapter the following would be helpful:

Acquaintance with a repertoire of activities that have therapeutic potential.

Access to a variety of clinical settings and patient/clients. Knowledge of the basic principles of therapeutic communication.

Methods and media and tools and techniques are the components, in varying combinations, of a therapeutic activities program. Methods and media will be discussed in this chapter; tools and techniques will have a chapter to themselves.

Media (Activities)

It is quite apparent from previous discussions that the primary media of occupational therapy are activities. The conditions under which activities become therapeutic for the individual have already been set out in detail in Chapter 4. Other considerations, however, that relate to external circumstances also affect the organization and administration of activities in therapeutic programs. No matter in which setting occupational therapy is practiced — clinic, hospital, nursing home, school, community center, prison, or the patient/client's home — a number of constraints are imposed on programs by environmental conditions; external rules, regulations, and policies; and the implicit but nonetheless pervasive value system operating in the setting. One such situation not uncommonly encountered is the limited space allocated to occupational therapy in plans for new hospital departments, regardless of the numbers of patients and the kinds of equipment needed. In many instances, particularly where treatment of physical disabilities is concerned, this reflects a value system that gives a low priority to a discipline dealing with quality of life, because such a discipline is neither essential in a life-saving sense nor "scientific" in a technological sense.

Activities and External Constraints

To meet patient/client needs within the limitations imposed by external conditions requires that activities be:

1. *Appropriate.* They should be appropriate not only in terms of meaning and relevance to the patient/client but also to the setting in which the activities programs are applied. It might be ideal, for instance, to install power tools for woodworking in a clinic treating a large number of injured workmen; but the physical structure of the clinic and its staffing patterns may preclude constant supervision, or, more of a problem still, the structure of the building may not meet required safety standards.

2. *Practical.* They should be practical, in the sense that they can be administered quickly and easily without laborious preparation, that they can be completed within the time frames imposed by the setting, and that they fit within budgetary restrictions. The decline in popularity of weaving as a therapeutic activity may be attributed in part to the time-consuming and laborious effort entailed in preparing the warp and threading the loom. Another reason may be the size and unwieldiness of the looms — which relate to the criterion of appropriateness as much as that of practicality.

3. *Versatile.* They should lend themselves, by virtue of their properties and characteristics, to a variety of processes, end products, and situations. A broad appeal, often related to current fad and fancy, across cultural, age, sex, and other differences also adds to the versatility of an activity.

An example of a very versatile activity, particularly in this day and age in our society, is cooking. The processes and end products are endless in their variety, ranging from the utilitarian fixing of a sandwich and the routines of preparing a family meal to the highest flights of haute cuisine, from pasting recipes in a scrapbook to the production of a cookbook with an exotic theme.

A most creative activity project at the tasting end was conceived for a group of young adults who needed to develop interpersonal and decision-making skills prior to returning to jobs in the community. In twos, they explored restaurants in the community serviced by the hospital and wrote their own version of a restaurant guide, having developed criteria and procedures for evaluation by group consensus. They also designed and produced a printed version, cover and all, allocating and organizing tasks with minimal direction from the therapist.

4. *Adaptable.* Activities should be adaptable to individual, and thus different, patient needs. The adaptable elements in activities are their properties and characteristics and the field of action.

The game of marabaraba, for instance, and indeed any game played with a board and checkers, lends itself to adaptation in many ways. In the case of the patient referred to in Chapter 4, the game was adapted to incorporate lower limb motion by use of greatly enlarged pieces, the introduction of wire hoops, an expanded area for the board, and location on the ground instead of on a table top. Many other physical adaptations are possible. For the individual lying flat in bed, this type of game can be played overhead with pieces (felt, Velcro-backed, or magnetic) that cling to the board, which is clamped in place to ensure correct positioning. The game may be placed vertically on an easel to ensure standing balance and shoulder and elbow motions. The pieces can be shaped in a number of ways to ensure particular kinds of finger function, or weighted for resistive motion. (See numerous articles and pictures in current and back issues of the *American Journal of Occupational Therapy* that describe other adapted activities.)

The field of action may also be modified in a number of ways. The setting may range from clinic, dayroom, or bedside to outdoors in the hospital grounds, from a quiet corner of a library to a recreation hall in which the game is set up in tournament style and rules are added for a laddering system that advances the ultimate winner to the top. The number of people can be varied from an intensely involved and isolated dyad through numerous combinations of persons to a large and vociferous group encompassing players and spectators. Adaptation of the explicit rules of the game is also possible. The game may end for one session when a specified number of pieces are captured, thus shortening and simplifying the process; the interaction between players may be prolonged by a challenge to return match; or a win may be determined by the best of a prearranged total of games.

Actual and Simulated Situations

Activities in a field of action are quite literally rehearsals for everyday living. Therefore, the more closely activities situations resemble the activities patterns in the real world, the better. In many instances activities can readily be introduced into the patient/client's day in patterns that approximate those that are socioculturally approved. Daily living skills such as eating and dressing can be practiced in most settings at appropriate times in real situations (even though institutional hours scarcely coincide with those of the real world). Similarly, leisure activities, among which are arts and crafts, pastimes, and hobbies selected for individual pleasure and gratification, lend themselves to administration in close approximation to actual situations.

However, because of the great range of patient/client needs, the variations in individual and sociocultural activities configurations, and the constraints inherent in the settings in which occupational therapy is administered, activities have for the most part to serve only as simulations of situations encountered in the real world. It is for this reason that the criteria of versatility and adaptability are so important. And it is also why arts and crafts, which fulfill these criteria more fully than most other kinds of activities, have played a dominant role in occupational therapy programs. It is necessary to examine only one craft, pottery, to realize the potential for an infinite number of structural variations designed to meet a number of different needs.

Imagine now an individual crouched in solitary absorption, raising a pot on a wheel. Inherent in this situation is intense involvement, self-expression, a creative outlet, satisfaction, and ultimately approval by others of a beautiful, tangible object. In another setting, four individuals sit around a table, each place neatly set out with appropriate materials, with a number of tools in the center for all to share. They concentrate intently on the therapist, who demonstrates step by step how to measure and cut out a ceramic tile — the setting and rules designed to facilitate interpersonal communication, which will in turn lead to completion of a set task. An attenuated assembly line — simulating conditions in the world of work — occupies a long room. Individuals work in clusters, each cluster being responsible for one stage in the process of manufacturing molded ceramic coffee mugs — pouring slip, unmolding, trimming, sanding, decorating, stacking the kiln. All clear away and clean up. A foreman allocates the jobs, checks on punctuality, and supervises the workers, while a general supervisor plans the overall project and checks on quality and quantity of production. There are sanctions for nonadherence to rules and material rewards for compliance (examples are tokens, credits toward a weekend pass, a movie, or dining out with the group). The therapist watches and intercedes only when necessary. Some individuals lead; most individuals follow, but have room for upward mobility as a reward for good performance. The end products are sold, and the profits are contributed to the patient government committee. In yet another situation, a young man with a splint on his hand rolls out and pinches clay into the shape of an ashtray as the therapist watches closely for substitute motions and signs of fatigue.

Needless to say, arts and crafts can be integrated into actual situations as well. An excellent example of how this can be done is an aftercare plan for a group of adolescent girls who were to live in a house in the community. The house needed extensive repair and redecoration, and the activities program encompassed painting, woodworking, sewing, decorative needlework, macramé, lampshade-making, furniture-refinishing, upholstery, textile design, linoprinting, and tile-setting. There were also heated discussions about themes, color schemes, styles, and designs for living. In this instance, the arts and crafts program not only cut across the boundaries of work, chore, leisure, social, and recreational activities but transcended them as a total experience in communal living.

The use of simulated situations is justified by the underlying assumption that learning can be transferred from one situation to another by generalization. Ideally in any activities program, provision is made to check whether this is in fact the case by giving activities assignments and following up on patient/client performance in actual situations. It goes almost without saying, for instance, that for a housewife with cardiac failure, no amount of practice in energy-saving techniques in the simulated kitchen of the occupational therapy clinic will suffice if she does not adapt her newly acquired skills to the kitchen in her own home and carry them through to other household activities.

Although simulations do have their place, it is important to bear in mind that arts and crafts or games or any other kinds of activities will be effective only if:

1. they have meaning and relevance to the patient/client;
2. their purpose is clear and acceptable to the patient/client, either as stages toward the attainment of activities health or as situations that are parallel to those in the real world;
3. there are enough elements of similarity between simulated and actual situations to make transfer of learning likely, whether it be to increasingly complex situations or to parallel situations.

As a general rule, actual situations should be selected, whenever possible, in preference to simulated situations. And there may be more actual situations available than one is aware of, even in a small clinic (see Chapter 6, Assignment 2, page 65). That artifice can be taken to ludicrous extremes is evidenced by the prevalent use of a plastic material as a substitute for meat when practice is needed in cutting with a knife. The color and texture of the plastic not only bear no resemblance to any known food, tasty or otherwise, but are an assault to the senses. And the danger of overdoing the arts and crafts is highlighted by the remark of one bright young student living in a wheelchair. As a member of a panel to discuss how rehabilitation helps the patient, he said of occupational therapy: "The underlying idea is great. But you people missed the boat when you gave us macramé belts to knot instead of a chance to make hamburgers in the kitchen!" A summary of a few typical situations, actual and simulated, cross-classified with chore, leisure-time, work-related, social, and recreational activities serves to clarify their relationships to each other (Table 5-1).

Methods
Methods are the procedures and processes by which activities are organized, integrated, and administered in therapeutic programs. These procedures and processes include:

1. *Selection.* Activities are selected on the basis of patient/client needs within the constraints of the particular setting in which the program

Table 5-1. A Summary of Typical Actual and Simulated Activities/Situations

	Actual* { "Real world" environment, rules, and/or time segments	Simulated* { Adapted or modified environment, rules, and/or time segments
Chores	Dressing and grooming, making bed, shopping	Grooming class, practicing getting in and out of dry bathtub, improving grip on practice board of variously shaped faucets and switches
Leisure	Hobbies and pastimes, expressive activities engaged in by individual choice and for individual gratification	Dance as communication, table games for hand-eye coordination
Work	Mail room help, typing, babysitting for staff (remuneration may be token rather than actual)	Pottery assembly line, woodworking
Social	Clubs, community action groups, family weekend outings	Group making ceramic tiles and sharing tools, family mural, monthly resident birthday celebration
Recreational	Sports, team games, matches, movies, concerts — outside the institution	Same activities within institutional constraints of time and setting

*All activities listed in this column are examples.

takes place. Needs are established by the collection and interpretation of data obtained from functional evaluations, case records, and activities histories; knowledge of individual and sociocultural activities configurations; and the patient/client's stated needs and wants. The selection of activities is made to facilitate attainment of a number of stated goals, which are based on patient/client needs and the constraints of the setting in which the program takes place. Alternative selections are an important part of the process, to allow for unexpected situational contingencies and changes in the patient/client's status.

2. *Structuring.* The activities selected are structured in ways that make them therapeutic. These include breakdown of each activity into manageable steps; integration with a systematic approach to management of dysfunction; decision on number and sequencing of activities to be incorporated into the program, with provision for making changes as the patient/client moves toward function; inclusion of visible means of checking progress; and, when necessary, adaptation or modification of activities and their field of action or the introduction of assistive devices, or both.

3. *Scheduling.* Each activity has to be integrated into the patient/client's daily schedule; one activity is dovetailed with another, time periods are allocated for each activity, and frequency and duration of each activities session are determined.

4. *Interaction.* The interaction between occupational therapist and patient/client is the cornerstone of the therapeutic process. As a specialist in therapeutic activities, the occupational therapist serves as a competence model in every interaction from the first interview onward. But the occupational therapist is also a facilitator. Outside each activities situation itself, the occupational therapist plans, organizes, evaluates progress, serves as an advocate for the patient/ client with professional colleagues and agencies or as a counselor with the family, and engages in a number of transactions with the patient/client in ways that are designed, step by step, to guide the individual toward independence in activities functioning. Because functioning includes not only activity performance per se but also the ability to plan, solve problems, make decisions, initiate action, and carry over skills to a number of different situations, the occupa-

tional therapist intervenes less and less as the patient/client does more and more with increasing confidence and a growing sense of competence.

Within each activities situation, the interaction between occupational therapist and patient/client varies with the individual's needs. For the patient withdrawn into a schizophrenic world, an intense, one-to-one relationship — the therapist a nurturing figure, recognizing and responding to the patient's dependency needs — may be the most effective beginning. On the other hand, for an office worker, whose activities routine includes typing for strengthening and coordination of fingers and wrist, the occupational therapist is a matter-of-fact but eagle-eyed supervisor who checks periodically to ensure correct positioning, watches the time carefully, and evaluates progress at the end of the session; and, in addition, encourages the intelligent, well-motivated individual to work on creative solutions for coping with daily chores at home. At the other extreme, the occupational therapist, having set up the activities situation, may remain at the periphery, delegating a number of leadership tasks to the patient/client and intervening only under predetermined conditions. This kind of interaction is apparent in the description of the ceramic assembly line on pages 50–51.

Determination of the patient/client's readiness for the acceptance of increasing responsibility is not simple. In our present state of knowledge, there are too few systematic links between behavior and performance to provide predictive criteria on which to base decisions. An illustration is provided in the case of Mrs. B, who played an unusually accurate game of tennis, was a productive member of the library committee, dressed with meticulous neatness, and was a superb craftswoman. During a particularly busy crafts session, the therapist directed her to fetch another length of leather lacing from the cupboard, to join to the piece that had run out while she was assembling a wallet. Half an hour later, when the bustle in the craft room had died down, the therapist found Mrs. B transfixed at the cupboard, face furrowed with anxiety, unable to decide which of two almost identical lengths would most closely match the one that needed joining.

In this instance, the underlying symptomatology had been glossed over by a deceptive competence. On the other hand, neither preconceptions based on clinical labeling nor a direct correlation between one kind of performance and another will serve any more accurately in the judgment of levels of functioning. The story of S emphasizes this point well.

S, a beautifully dressed, delicate 12-year-old, was brought to the prevocational evaluation unit by her distraught parents. Both successful professionals, they were still unable to accept that their only child had been labeled severely mentally retarded and therefore ineducable. S, neat as a new pin, liked nothing better than to clean and tidy up and so became acquainted with the old, creaky mimeograph machine. Her interest in the stencils, as she removed them carefully and efficiently for machine cleaning, prompted me to wonder whether she could learn to fasten them into place correctly. And, after painstaking, step-by-step practice, she succeeded — upside down, reverse, and all. So adept did she become that one day I called from across the other end of the room: "S, when you have the stencil in place, roll off 100 copies." I looked up and caught the expression on her face — like a puppy that had been beaten. Then it dawned on me — she could operate the machine, but the concept of 100 completely eluded her, because she could count only to 10. This particular story has a happy ending. When I told her that 100 meant a one, zero, zero side by side, she set the dial correctly and finished the job.

By the same token, underestimation of the patient/client's capabilities and potential for change is equally undesirable. As was established in Chapter 4, the will to learn is elicited when effort is required. And it is a matter of common observation that individuals tend to rise to the occasion, reinforcing Bruner's contention that situations have their own demand value. This is perhaps most vividly illustrated by the behavior of a group of patients in one of the back wards of a mental hospital. When a group of smartly turned out occupational therapy students visited, it was remarkable how many of the shrunken, unkempt, empty-eyed old men automatically straightened up, made ineffectual dabs at their uncombed hair, and tugged at nonexistent collars and ties.

In the reciprocity of the interaction, the perceptions, attitudes, and feelings of the occupational therapist can either facilitate or hold back progress toward independence in functioning for the patient/client. One of the most prevalent expectations — that patient/client progress will follow a neat sequence of orderly steps provided that certain formulas for action are followed — paves the way for frustration and disappointment on both sides. The development of independent functioning takes for the most part an uneven course, marked occasionally by encouraging leaps, with plateaus of quiescence, and even with regression (perhaps when expectations are too high or when achievement arouses anxiety about inability to respond to higher expectations). This recognition is the first step in establishing realistic guideposts for progress. The road to patient/client independence may also be blocked, all too often quite unwittingly, by the occupational therapist's personal needs, one of which is to retain the kind of control that is sanctioned under the guise of "helping."

Modes of interaction involve both verbal and nonverbal communication. Since much of the occupational therapy emphasis is on "doing," a large and significant part of the interaction between therapist and patient/client is nonverbal. However, with the high value placed on verbal facility as an interpersonal skill in our society, all too often many of the nuances of nonverbal communication are lost in an overlay of conversational gambits that are at times irrelevant and even countertherapeutic. The concrete evidence of achievement inherent in the activities situation may be far more telling than a number of mechanical phrases — such as "That's nice," "Very good," "Fine" — that accompany every action and are meant to be encouraging, whether the results are good, bad, or indifferent.

It is in the area of interaction that the clinical skills of the occupational therapist are called into play, skills that are more than the sum of knowledge of theoretical concepts and the ability to select and organize appropriate activities. These clinical skills require sensitivity to and awareness of patient/client needs, a fine attunement to the subtlest cues provided by the patient/client, ability to interpret those cues accurately, and a wholesome respect both for the uniqueness of each individual and for the shared human potential for change. Therapeutic communication is a study in itself. Hein [32] and Ruesch [62] offer valuable guidelines for the helping professional.

The detailed examination of methods and media has shown how activities are used for therapeutic purposes. The aids to adaptation, organization, and administration of therapeutic activities — tools and techniques — await discussion in the next chapter.

Assignments to Examine Activities in Terms of Criteria for Therapeutic Potential

1. In the clinics known to you, or visited, list the activities used that fulfill all the criteria for defining them as therapeutic.
2. List all the ways of adapting activities that you have observed. What other potential for adaptation — when you look at properties, characteristics, and field of action — do they have?
3. a. Consider the activities you have so far identified as being characteristic of your own way of life. Which of them, even though not used in any clinic you have observed, would lend themselves to use as therapeutic agents? Why?
   b. Consider in the same way activities that are characteristic of individuals quite different from you.
4. Make a list (without considering any external constraints) of activities that would have meaning and relevance for a number of patient/clients, each of whom you have selected from a different age group and socioeconomic background, and each of whom has different physical or psychosocial problems, or both. Reduce the list in each instance to those activities that are also (1) adaptable, (2) versatile, and (3) practical. Finally, list those that have a combination of all the qualities needed to make them therapeutically useful.

6. Tools and Techniques

In addition to what has already been required for previous chapters, the reader should be familiar with (1) the structure and function of a selection of devices, splints, and other kinds of tools and equipment used in occupational therapy; (2) a variety of clinical environments; and (3) a selection of studies that examine transfer and retention of learning in both children and adults.

Both tools and techniques are at the disposal of the occupational therapist to facilitate the appropriate use of activities for therapeutic purposes.

Tools

These are defined, in Bruner's sense [8], as amplifiers of human action and encompass:

1. *Equipment.* Equipment includes specially designed apparatus and devices that assist function or compensate for absent function, or labor-saving and convenience gadgets obtainable as standard merchandise. Examples of equipment range from wheelchairs, splints, prostheses, Braille watches, bathroom rails, and pocket calculators to universal cuffs, rocker knives, jar openers, and long-handled reachers. Some of the most efficient items of equipment are home-made devices of astonishing simplicity, such as a length of wood set with four nails hammered halfway in at one end to lock over an old-fashioned faucet — a boon to a housewife with early morning stiffness in her arthritic wrists and fingers, who can now lever the faucet open with shoulder abduction and elbow flexion. Another example is even more ingenious — the use of texture-matched tags stapled

like laundry labels in an inconspicuous but accessible spot, to coordinate outfits for a blind business executive living alone. Other items of equipment are designed and constructed by the occupational therapist and include splints and devices to aid function, such as cuffs to hold writing and eating utensils.

Equipment may be applied or attached to:
1. the patient/client, e.g., splints, slings, prostheses, weighted cuffs, functional devices.
2. objects in the environment, e.g., bath rails, jar opener attached to kitchen shelf, armrests for chair.
3. activities apparatus, e.g., padded grip for printing press lever, easel for checkerboard, pulley and weight for vertical sanding block.

2. *Environments.* These consist of physical settings, people, and objects. Occupational therapy is carried out in a variety of *settings* but need not be confined to the space formally allocated to its operations. The game of marabaraba (see Chapter 4) is moved to a path outside the tiny occupational therapy department. An unfrequented corner of a pediatric floor is an area admirably suited to a game of sedentary balloon volleyball for a group of children recovering from extensive burns. The dayroom of a unit is a good place to practice social skills with coffee, cake, and a demonstration of beauty products for a group of women for whom the state institution is home, while the gymnasium, preempted for an hour, becomes a ballroom for elderly men and women with Parkinson's disease. In good weather, the hospital grounds, with their lawns and trees, are the best possible setting for the intricate needlework project that is the means of communication between a therapist and a withdrawn young mother; and the gift shop run by the women's auxiliary offers a practical and realistic way to help an uncoordinated adolescent cope with the hazards of shopping — communicating his needs to the salesperson, negotiating the narrow aisles cluttered with merchandise projecting from the shelves, selecting and carrying an item to the cash desk, taking money from a purse, and gathering up change and package.

The *interpersonal environment* with its rules for interaction can be varied as much as the physical setting. At one extreme the occupational therapist and patient/client may be isolated in a secluded area from which extraneous stimuli have been deliberately excluded, while at the other extreme the patient/client may be at the center of a large and vociferous group (the marabaraba game again).

The *objects* in the environment encompass (1) those that may be peripheral to the activities situation — such as the furnishings of a room — and (2) those that are deliberately incorporated into the field of action — such as tools, a special arrangement of chairs, or the merchandise in the hospital gift shop described on page 60.

In most cases environments are preselected and structured, but there are instances, given the appropriate milieu, where the selection of environment and indeed an activities "happening" can occur quite spontaneously, as the following episode illustrates:

It has been more than usually hectic in the occupational therapy department. Walking along the glassed-in corridor I glimpse the inner court, enticingly empty — a good place to munch apple and cheese and unwind from the morning's tensions. I enjoy the coolness of the stone bench and the marvelous patterns formed by the multicolored pebbles on the ground. In wanders R, fair hair disheveled, pale eyes dreamy and distant. Diffidently, he asks if he may join me. A social overture from R — usually so withdrawn, beset with his inner demons — how can I refuse? He crouches down beside the bench, poking among the pebbles with a stick. We sit in companionable silence for a while. Then — "Look at the colors" — his eyes still fixed on the pebbles — "lovely swirly patterns — just stones — and these tiny little plants coming up between them — and they're alive." "Yes," I say, "isn't it incredible? Pushing up for survival among the stones, tiny as they are." He looks up at that, dreamy film gone, and smiles. We talk on, about the trees fringing the courtyard, the number of birds that come to visit, growing plants as a hobby, bird-watching. Several other young people have drifted in, and we are now deeply into environment, pollution, and ecology; some are professorial like R, others contribute their opinions in the pithy language of the streets. "Hey, man," says S, "we could make our own ecology group — that ____ pile back of the OT could be cleared up for a start." The lunch break has moved fast. In trots B, cute face plastered with rouge, deep blue eyes fringed with improbable spikes, platform shoes clattering on the pebbles. She looks at me anxiously. "Is this a special group?" (We use group activities a great deal in the hospital.) "Yes, it's a special group for special people. Come join us for the time we have left."

3. *Time.* Time amplifies human action in that a number of repetitions over time are required to ensure that:

   1. learning is integrated enough to ensure carry-over to appropriate situations
   2. physical changes, such as building up of endurance, can take place
   3. interpersonal relationships can be established
   4. newly acquired skills can be applied and tested in a variety of situations.

Time, as has been discussed in Chapter 3, is also an important tool for the organization of activities in socioculturally acceptable patterns, thus defining reality. In many instances, an individual's chief problem may be, for a variety of clinical reasons, inability to budget time effectively. This includes not only underactivity, but the kind of overactivity that can turn a period of free time into a fearsome experience for an anxiety-ridden individual.

A device that uses a time frame for organizing activities is a simple one and familiar to all students — the weekly printed schedule. It is useful simply as a tool of organization, but it may also require of the individual an increasing assumption of responsibility, e.g., in making selections from a repertoire of choices, solving problems of clashes and conflicts, and budgeting time realistically. The "musts" and electives as well as free periods, meal breaks, and the unwritten time to be allocated for preparation, travel, and other contingencies apply as much to general activities patterns as to those of the student.

Techniques
Techniques are those procedures that are derived from theoretical propositions or are based on an empirical approach. As indicated in

Chapter 4 (see page 37), there are numerous theories about human function and dysfunction and numerous treatment approaches arising from them. To be incorporated into occupational therapy programs, it is important that such procedures:

1. relate to the physical and psychological needs of the individual
2. "make sense" in an activities-related system of intervention
3. dovetail with those activities procedures and situations that can successfully be administered within the constraints of a particular setting.

For the occupational therapist to select the most appropriate technique requires sufficient knowledge of the theoretical concepts and the methods advocated to answer the following questions:

1. What does the proponent have to say about the nature of the human condition?
2. How does the proponent differentiate a functional from a dysfunctional individual?
3. What stages of development lead to function or dysfunction?
4. By what mechanisms does change from dysfunction toward function take place?
5. In what time period is change expected to take place?

(A work sheet for this kind of analytical look at theoretical approaches will be found in Appendix 4. See also Assignment 4 at the end of Chapter 4.)

An example of a carefully documented, step-by-step treatment method based on empirical observation and a theoretical rationale is that advanced by Brunnstrom [11]. Her fundamental premise is that recovery from hemiplegia in adults follows a sequence that parallels the ontogenetic development of neuromuscular control — from preponderance of reflex activity, through linked patterns of movement, toward ultimate dissociation from synergies, and finally voluntary control. At the basis of treatment are two assumptions: (1) that sensory input can influence motor input; and (2) that recovery can be hastened by first harnessing the mechanisms present in the existing level of function/ dysfunction (e.g., reflex activity), and then incorporating them with sensory input and feedback into a series of facilitation techniques, which lead toward the next stage of recovery.

The techniques for evaluating level of function/dysfunction and for facilitating change in the direction from dysfunction toward function are precisely and clearly described by Brunnstrom. It is for the occupational therapist to examine the method and ask if it meshes appropriately with an activities frame of reference. One of the crucial determinations to be made, assuming that Brunnstrom's propositions "make sense," is at which stage of recovery it is possible to begin occupational therapy. Is Stage 1, flaccidity, the point at which the needs of the patient can be met by incorporation of an activities program? Perhaps — if the unaffected side is used to facilitate associated responses that will influence the development of tone in the muscles of the affected side. On the other hand, if occupational therapy incorporates bimanual activities when spasticity has developed, what then will be the effect on muscle tone? How does this consideration affect the planning, organization, and administration of activities, when one bears in mind that these activities also must have meaning and relevance to the patient/client?

In another example, two theoretical approaches have been combined to serve as an underlying rationale. It is apparent from the title of the protocol for an activities group in a psychiatric clinic (Appendix 5) that Erikson's view of psychosocial development [20] is one of the theoretical approaches selected. The other approach relates to theories about group process, particularly those that examine the effects of leadership styles on group dynamics [44]. In the protocol, the dynamics of the activities group have been linked to Erikson's description of the characteristic features of one particular stage of psychosocial development. Criteria for admission to and movement out of the group have been determined on the basis of behavioral indexes that reveal attainment of prior developmental stages and readiness for further movement. Since this method, unlike Brunnstrom's, was applied directly to an activities base, the activities selected fall neatly into place and reflect the sociocultural activities configurations of the group.

Techniques, together with activities and the tools for amplifying human action, are the instruments by which an individual is helped to a state of activities health. The methods adopted by the occupational therapist ensure that those instruments are best suited to the psychological and physical needs of the individual, and that they serve their purpose in an orderly, controlled progression from easy to difficult, simple to complex, assisted to resisted, minimally stressful to maximally stressful — on the way toward functional independence for the patient/client.

Assignments to Take a Closer Look at the Tools and Techniques of Occupational Therapy

1. Make your own reference book from clippings or copies of articles, diagrams, and advertisements that appear in journals of occupational therapy, journals in allied fields, and sketches in suppliers' catalogues. Classify and index the information in a way that will be helpful to both therapist and patient/client seeking a ready guide to the kinds of equipment and materials available as self-help devices and splints. Add drawings and descriptions of ingenious devices you have seen in clinics or of those you may have designed or constructed yourself.

   Read Zimmerman's article "Devices: Development and Direction" [72].

2. Whenever you visit a clinic, make notes of the potential for using environments other than the space formally assigned. Consider even long-distance therapeutic situations — e.g., a phone call from a patient who, in great trepidation, had to negotiate a subway alone but arrived safely at her destination, or letters to and from patient/clients. (Little M, dying of a congenital and irremediable cardiac condition, received a picture-letter from her vacationing occupational therapist, in which was enclosed a small bag of sea sand and tiny shells glued to the pages between funny sketches of the fishermen and bathing belles — a gesture that eased a little of the pain and grief of dying for her and her parents.) Read "Writing Therapy: A New Approach

to Treatment and Training," Chapter 9 in *Short-Term Psychotherapy and Structured Behavior Change* [54] , and see if these concepts can be applied in occupational therapy.

3. In using time as a tool for organizing and administering activities, look for ways of answering these questions:

a. *Frequency.* How *often* is it necessary for a process or procedure to be repeated to ensure that learning takes place and will be retained?

b. *Duration.* Over how long a period does the process or procedure have to be repeated?

c. Under which conditions does repetition integrate learning?

d. Under which conditions does repetition extinguish learning?

7. Principles of Occupational Therapy

A number of general principles of occupational therapy follow from a point of view centered on activities both as therapeutic agents and as beacons of healthy functioning. These principles, which are applicable to any form of intervention for any patient/client, relate to the four stages that characterize the total occupational therapy process. These four stages are: *Initial Assessment, Planning, Implementation,* and *Termination.*

Stage 1. Initial Assessment

Stage 1 is designed for two purposes: (1) to establish patient/client needs; and (2) to establish whether occupational therapy can help meet these needs.

The processes and procedures used in the initial assessment are directed to answering the following questions:

Who is this individual who has come for help?

What is this individual's activities configuration in terms of past and present experiences and future wishes?

What is the sociocultural activities configuration of the group to which this individual belongs?

What are the physical, intellectual, emotional, and interpersonal skills required to perform these activities in ways that are individually satisfying and socioculturally acceptable?

Which of these skills does the individual have?

Which of these skills have never been developed?

Which of these skills has the individual lost, temporarily or permanently?

How long have these skills been lost or unavailable?

What are the possibilities for (1) regaining lost skills, (2) compensating or substituting for lost skills, (3) achieving new skills?

What are the probabilities, given realistic constraints, of regaining these
skills?

In order to answer these questions, it is clear that the occupational
therapist requires special assessment tools as well as special emphases in
gathering data, even if evaluation tools or findings from other disciplines
are incorporated for use. The activities history referred to in Chapter 4
and activities situations structured to elicit specific kinds of activities-
related behavior, whether it be as varied as leadership skill or performance of thumb and finger prehension, are two of the most valuable,
but as yet not systematically applied, approaches to assessment of
levels of functioning [12, 16]. In the realms of physical dysfunction, a
functional evaluation — that is, an assessment of the basic patterns of
motion required for functioning in day-to-day living — is much more to
the point for occupational therapy than measurement of isolated ranges
of joint motion and strength of individual muscles. Indeed, goniometry
and muscle testing are useful only in as far as they can be directly cor-
related with an assessment of functional level in the skills necessary for
performance of activities. Guarding against indiscriminate use of evaluation tools and overzealous accumulation of data is important for effective assessment.

Since prognoses and projections have to be made, it is necessary not
only to gather data but to interpret them. An interpretation that leads
to determination of patient/client needs based on strengths and liabilities, general life-style, and wishes and desires also permits the decision
to be made as to whether occupational therapy is able to provide assistance in meeting those needs. The principles of occupational therapy
emerge as follows:

1. Begin every occupational therapy program with an initial assessment.
2. Select carefully from existing data or methods of obtaining data to
   ensure that information about the activities needs of the patient/
   client will be obtained in the most economical way.
3. Correlate and interpret data in terms of patient/client strengths
   and liabilities as they relate to skills needed for activities functioning.
4. Determine, in the light of assessment of patient/client needs, whether
   occupational therapy is able to assist in meeting those needs.

Stage 2. Planning

Stage 2 involves:

1. defining goals for meeting patient/client needs
2. establishing priorities in the case of multiple goals
3. designing a program that will lead the patient/client, step by step, toward attainment of the goals

The design of the program encompasses selection of activities and their field of action, selection of appropriate tools and techniques, breakdown of activities processes into manageable steps, adaptation of activities (if necessary), and scheduling, not only for activities per se but for sessions directed to evaluating progress (see Chapters 5 and 6). Into the design is built provision for changes in program, either because of changes in patient/client condition or because of changes in external circumstances. The establishment of realistic goals requires of the occupational therapist the ability to predict in some measure the results of following an advocated method and the length of time required for those results to occur. Principles for planning include the following:

1. Establish goals that not only meet patient/client needs but can realistically be carried out within the constraints of the therapeutic situation.
2. Establish both long-range overall goals and short-term goals as attainable steps toward reaching the long-term goals (at times these may merge).
3. Select activities for each short-term goal that have meaning and relevance for the patient/client.
4. Select activities as alternatives to be held in reserve in case of changes.
5. Structure activities situations in ways that arouse and harness the will to learn.
6. Select and schedule activities situations that are as close as possible to situations in the real world.
7. Incorporate the simplest and the least number of adaptations possible to ensure maximal function.
8. Use the simplest and the least amount of equipment possible to effect maximal function.

9. Schedule activities with sufficient frequency of repetition and duration to ensure integration of learning.
10. Schedule specific periods for evaluation of progress and subsequent adjustment or modification of program.
11. Establish conditions for interaction with patient/client (e.g., frequency of teaching; kinds of intervention, directive or nondirective; closeness; ways of reinforcing desired behaviors; ways of evaluating progress; delegation of parts of program to others; incorporation of others into program, as in group activities or with family).

Stage 3. Implementation

Implementation is the carrying out of the occupational therapy plan, which includes structuring of activities situations, instruction in activities procedures, interaction with patient/client, observation of precautions, observation of patient/client performance and attendant behaviors, and evaluation of progress. The plan is adjusted according to patient/client responses and modified according to step-by-step progress toward attainment of goals. Principles for implementation are:

1. Prepare activities before start of session, observing precautions for patient/client safety (e.g., clear working area, careful placement of sharp implements, adequate lighting, nonskid surfaces, heat-proof holders).
2. Prepare activities in their field of action to ensure the use of predetermined setting and correct positioning of patient/client; ensure that equipment, interpersonal field, and objects are arranged as planned.
3. Break activities down into manageable steps, explaining the relationship of one step to another.
4. When instructing, explain in ways comprehensible to the patient/client, checking to see that each step has been mastered before proceeding to the next.
5. When demonstrating, make sure your starting position is the same as the patient/client's (sit when patient/client is sitting; stand when it is desired that patient/client stand; face same way as patient/client).

6. Check, at appropriate intervals, to ensure maintenance of correct positioning and standard of performance.
7. Watch for signs of fatigue or stress or unusual behavior, and respond accordingly, either suspending activity or adjusting the situation as required.
8. Graduate amount of support and assistance given according to patient/client responses.
9. Follow conditions for interaction established in the plan.
10. Incorporate a visible means for checking progress (e.g., score in a game, recording of time taken to perform, number of knots achieved toward completion in a macramé belt, completion of an end product, number of pounds of weight lifted, tokens earned) in the steps of each activity.
11. Prepare patient/client for continuity of program by outlining plan for the following session or soliciting suggestions from patient/client, when ready to contribute.

Stage 4. Termination
Tapering off and ending a patient/client program in preparation for independent carry-over of newly acquired skills into the real world of day-to-day living is of such crucial importance that *termination* is designated as a separate stage.

Under ideal conditions, goals should be reached in a predictable period of time, so that termination plans, including preparation of the patient/client for separation by an increasing number of assignments at home and in the community, are incorporated well in advance. Unfortunately, particularly in institutional settings, a number of externally imposed conditions often preclude such planning, much less follow-up of patient/client progress after termination. Sometimes the intercession of the occupational therapist with a well-considered plan may "buy time" for the patient/client, or result in referral to another agency for the period of transition. But in all events, if occupational therapy is to fulfill its promise for the patient/client, the stage of termination, and the principles that apply, must be considered as an integral part of the occupational therapy process.

Table 7-1. Summary of the Occupational Therapy Process.

Time Frame	Principles	Interaction	
		Therapist	Patient/ Client
1 day to 1 week	**Stage 1. Initial Assessment**		
	1. Begin all programs with initial assessment	F	M–F
	2. Select suitable data-gathering methods	F	
	3. Correlate all data and interpret	F	
	4. Determine patient/client's needs	F	
	Initial assessment consists of:		
	Data collection	F	M–F
	Interpretation of data	F	M
Variable	**Stage 2. Planning**		
	1. Establish goals, both long-term and short-term	F	M–F
	2. Select activities on the basis of established criteria	F	M–F
	3. Structure activities in a field of action	F	F
	4. Incorporate adaptations and equipment with discrimination and restraint	F	M–F
	5. Schedule according to criteria that will assure therapeutic administration	F	M–F
	6. Establish conditions for interaction	F	
	Planning consists of:		
	Definition of goals	F	M–F
	Establishment of priorities	F	M–F
	Design of a program	F	M–F
Variable	**Stage 3. Implementation**		
	1. Prepare activities situation as determined in plan	F	M–F
	2. Instruct according to a methodical sequence of steps	F	

M = minimal participation; F = full participation; M–F = minimal to full shared participation.

Table 7-1 (Continued)

Time Frame	Principles	Interaction	
		Therapist	Patient/ Client
	3. Check correct positioning and standard of performance periodically	F	
	4. Graduate amount of supervision and interaction	M–F	
	5. Follow conditions for interaction as determined in plan	F	M–F
	6. Incorporate a means for checking progress	F	
	7. Prepare patient/client for each required step	F	M–F
	Implementation consists of:		
	Structuring of activities situations	F	M–F
	Instruction in activities procedures	F	M–F
	Interaction with patient/client	M–F	M–F
	Observation of precautions	F	
	Observation of patient/client performance and attendant behaviors	F	
	Evaluation of progress	F	M–F
Variable	**Stage 4. Termination**		
	1. Prepare patient/client for termination	F	F
	2. Establish links with family, other individuals, and community agencies	F	M–F
	3. Prepare activities plan for daily living at home	M	F
	4. Arrange for follow-up	F	F
	Termination consists of:		
	Tapering off program for ultimate independent or near-independent functioning in home and community	M	F
	Follow-up	F	F

The principles for termination are:

1. Prepare patient/client for termination of program by indicating possible termination date (at times in consultation with the therapeutic team), acknowledging and dealing with separation anxiety as needed.
2. Assign as many activities requiring near-independent or independent functioning as possible, preferably in the home or community.
3. Establish links with the family and other individuals important to patient/client to ensure support for carry-over of activities into the home.
4. Establish links with agencies in the community that can be of assistance to the patient/client.
5. Prepare, with the patient/client, family, and other individuals a plan for a day-to-day activities program that will be personally satisfying as well as socioculturally acceptable.
6. Arrange for follow-up reports, or other contacts to review functioning, at regular intervals.

An alternative to steps 3, 4, and 5 would be to refer the patient/client, with a proposed activities plan, to a community agency or community therapist for furtherance of independent or near-independent functioning in the home and community.

Besides these general principles, which serve as a framework for operation, there are specific principles that arise out of specific situations and specific theoretical approaches. All have to be integrated into the occupational therapy program. The patient/client participates in each stage as fully as physical, emotional, and intellectual capacities allow. Table 7-1 (pp. 72–73) summarizes the stages of the occupational therapy process, the principles that apply to each, and the points at which active participation by the patient/client, ranging from minimal contributions to complete independence from the therapist, is possible.

Assignments to Practice the Principles of Occupational Therapy

1. Teach yourself a new skill from written instructions. Record your responses and reactions as you go through the learning process and

the time taken to learn the skill. Note the modifications you would make in recommending this method of learning to another individual. Now that you have mastered the skill, analyze step by step the procedure you would use to impart it to other individuals in age groups, sociocultural groups, and levels of intelligence different from your own.

2. Practice teaching a fellow student or colleague a skill that is familiar to you but that you do not particularly enjoy. Ask for comments and suggestions from your pupil at the end of the teaching session. This may also be done with the addition of a group of observers who contribute their comments at the end of the session.

3. Try out a number of different ways of introducing yourself and an activity to an individual who:
   a. is considerably older than you
   b. is much younger than you
   c. finds it difficult to communicate verbally
   d. has some form of sensory deprivation
   e. appears to you to be superior
   Compare your methods with those of your fellow students or colleagues.

4. Plan programs for as many patient/clients as you can, even though you are not likely to participate in the implementation.

5. Take every opportunity you can in the clinic to practice applying the principles of occupational therapy in a systematic way. Don't forget the termination plan!

II. Clinical Application

Three different individuals, with different problems, will help to illustrate how the principles of occupational therapy, based on a point of view centered on activities, can be translated into clinical practice.

The narrative style that follows is not typical of case-history writing; it has been deliberately chosen to lend substance and spirit to Mrs. B, P, and Mr. S. For we all know there is far more to any individual than is revealed by a collection of carefully assembled facts, even when they are accompanied by interpretations of their significance.

In each instance, after a full description of the patient/client and information that would usually come from an initial assessment, there are instructions for procedure. For Mrs. B (Case 1), the procedure is outlined step by step in great detail, following the principles set out in Chapter 7. For the other two, the procedure is based on the guidelines given for Mrs. B, requiring, of course, amendments and adaptations as appropriate. The key word *consider* draws attention to information that is particularly important as a basis for planning and implementation. *Notes* give information in addition to that found in case histories.

A number of brief case histories, which can serve as a further basis for practicing those procedures leading to clinical application, appear after the three major cases.

8. Case 1. Mrs. B

Appearance at First Interview

Mrs. B is a tiny, trim 58-year-old housewife. She looks younger than her years, despite streaks of gray in her dark hair, which is drawn back into a neat bun. Even with obvious spasticity in her right upper limb and a slight limp, she moves with an unusually erect carriage. Her eyes are large and brilliant, her face is unlined; but there is a perceptible droop at the corner of her mouth. While she is conversing the droop is accentuated, particularly during times when she struggles for an elusive word, frowning intently and testing several introductory syllables before finding the right one. Speech is thick but quite intelligible. Movements are slow and laborious. Her impatience shows occasionally as she playfully slaps her right hand, which does not perform as quickly and deftly as she would like.

Mrs. B was transferred from a general hospital to a rehabilitation center four months after the onset of a stroke, which has left her with a right residual hemiplegia. Besides occupational therapy, she was referred for physical therapy and speech therapy.

Background Data

Mrs. B lives in a third-floor walk-up, four-room apartment in an old house in a predominantly Black neighborhood with her husband, age 56, who is a truck driver. They have two children, a daughter and a son. The daughter, age 24, is a college graduate, is married, has one child, and lives in the South. The son, who has just completed college at 22, has a job as a reporter for a small-town newspaper. He is unmarried and lives about 40 miles away from his parents' home. The youngest, a son age 19, was killed in cross fire from a gang fight two weeks before Mrs. B had the stroke.

General Style of Living

Mrs. B is what might be termed a reluctant housewife. She is not particularly interested in household activities, including cooking, but has always kept her home "nice and clean; you can eat off the floor." She cuts cooking to a minimum. When her husband is away she eats very little. Breakfast out of a cereal box, lunch a simple sandwich, and a TV dinner are more the rule than the exception. Her husband, however, is a hearty eater and she feels it incumbent on her to take more interest in food preparation when he is at home. She considers it fortunate that her husband helps a great deal with the cooking and other household chores. Her chief tasks are bedmaking, washing dishes, setting the table, doing the laundry, dusting, and light cleaning for daily maintenance of the apartment.

Her own person is meticulously neat. She dresses simply and uses no make-up. She likes to get up early, shower, and dress immediately and get household chores over as soon as possible. She says she has been brought up to do her duty properly without complaining, even if she doesn't like what she does. Her father was a Baptist minister, and both she and her husband are regular churchgoers. They also participate in the social life emanating from the church, which has included group outings, picnics, travel, lectures, and Bible classes, mostly at weekends.

Her husband is a long-distance truck driver, so he is away from home at intervals, with as much as a week off between trips. She says, not without a twist of humor, that he gets under her feet when he is around, but he also helps with shopping, carrying heavy packages of household supplies upstairs for her, and cooking, which he greatly enjoys. He also enjoys watching TV variety and talk shows and boxing and basketball matches, and occasionally takes a turn at the basketball court at the park a few blocks away. They both go to bed early — before 10:30 P.M. — unless they are going to a church social.

Mr. B earns a "decent" salary, which enables them to live comfortably though simply. Both living children got through college with scholarships and part-time work. Their youngest son had been a promising athlete but had not accepted any of the several scholarships available to him. He had been working as a guitarist in a rock band at the time of his death.

The children and grandchild occasionally visit with the Bs, but the family communicate mainly by telephone, regularly on the part of the daughter, less frequently on the part of the son. The youngest son lived at home, but apparently because of his erratic hours he participated very little in daily family life. (Mrs. B is still very emotional about her son's death, so questioning has been kept to a minimum.) Mrs. B has few friends other than the families she is acquainted with through church activities. A neighbor's daughter, age 16, pops in several times a week to chat, especially when Mrs. B is alone. Mrs. B considers that she lives a quiet life, "where nothing much happens," except for the daily fear that she may be the next victim of a mugging, or worse.

Activities History

Mrs. B states that she was always a quiet and obedient child, unlike her two younger sisters, who were "regular tomboys." She never liked to get her pretty clothes dirty and was not interested in games involving physical activity. She cannot remember any favorite playthings, even dolls, and never wanted particularly to have a pet animal. All she has loved, and still does, are "books, books, and more books." Her face lights up as she recounts that she was a top pupil in English, and that she will read anything from stories of true romance to the Bible. Her scholastic record was so good that she obtained a Merit scholarship for college; however, her father died when she was in her second year, leaving her mother and two young sisters penniless. So she went to work as a packer in a perfume factory and stayed for 13 years, even after her sisters had begun working to support themselves and their mother. Besides work, her activities consisted of help with household chores, churchgoing, teaching at Sunday school, and reading. At the age of 32, shortly after her mother's death, she married, somewhat beneath her, she considers, because her husband barely managed to complete high school and is not interested in anything to do with "brain work."

Mrs. B continued her lifelong involvement in reading. She states she borrows books — mostly romantic novels — from the bookmobile of the public library, which parks at the nearby school once a week. Sometimes while shopping at the supermarket she will stop at nearby thrift shops and browse among the paperbacks, and she also picks up bargains at garage sales and fund-raising events at the church.

Physical Assessment

General Functioning

Mrs. B moves slowly and laboriously, but her sitting and standing balance is good. She walks with a slight limp, dragging her right foot. As she walks, the right upper limb is maintained in a position of flexion and adduction of the shoulder, partial flexion of the elbow, partial pronation of the forearm, and flexion of the wrist and fingers. She has some voluntary motion of the right upper limb, but can use it only as a gross assist, because movements are linked in synergies. Hand function consists of voluntary mass grasp, which she is able to release voluntarily by concentrating very hard. Her right side is dominant, but she has good coordination and dexterity on the left. Erect posture is well maintained; head is held in midline.

Motor Assessment

RIGHT UPPER LIMB. Motions are locked in flexion and extension synergies when voluntary motion is attempted. In both synergies wrist and fingers are flexed.

Passive range of motion. This is minimally limited in shoulder flexion, abduction, and external rotation, with pain in the final degrees of motion.

Active range of motion

Flexion Synergy			Extension Synergy	
Partial	Elevation	Shoulder girdle		
Full	Retraction			
Full	Hyperextension	Shoulder	Full	Adduction
Partial	Abduction		Full	Flexion
Partial	External rotation			
Full	Flexion	Elbow	Partial	Extension
Partial	Supination	Forearm	Partial	Pronation

<u>Spasticity</u>. Spasticity is present in elbow, wrist, and finger flexors.

HEAD, NECK, AND TRUNK. No spasticity was detected. There is full, active range of motion in neck and trunk rotation and trunk and neck forward flexion and extension. Ranges of motion of lateral flexion of neck and trunk are a few degrees short of full.

Sensory Assessment

RIGHT UPPER LIMB. Position sense and kinesthetic awareness are absent in shoulder and elbow.
   Tactile sensation is intact.

OCULAR PURSUIT. Ocular pursuit is within normal limits. Visual scanning is slow but accurate. There is no field neglect.

Integrated Functioning

Mrs. B is cooperative and anxious to do well. She has a tendency to drive herself beyond her physical limitations. She shows signs of fatigue long before she admits she is tired but is relieved when the therapist calls activity to a halt. She concentrates well and grasps instructions quickly. At times she has difficulty in correcting errors, even when she has recognized them herself. Memory appears to be unaffected.

She has a mild expressive aphasia. Any reference to her deceased son produces a marked emotional reaction — her eyes fill with tears, and her voice trembles. Since her admission to the hospital, she has cut herself off from current events, keeping away from newspapers and news broadcasts. She is independent in all self-care activities, maintaining an exquisitely neat appearance, and she has shown initiative and creativity in solving problems related to coping with tasks one-handed. In her eagerness to perform well and quickly, she tends to neglect her affected side. As she says: "I forget all about it!"

The Occupational Therapy Program

Initial Assessment	Notes
1. From the activities history and description of life-style, list the activities that Mrs. B:	*(Organization of data)*
a. carries out daily b. performs frequently (less than daily but more than once weekly) c. engages in occasionally	What other information would be useful and helpful? E.g., how Mrs. B feels about a predominantly "unexciting" life. What she would like to do best, if she could choose.
Draw up a timetable of a typical week in Mrs. B's life, coding activities by color (or in some other way) that would indicate the activities Mrs. B perceives as:	
d. important but not necessarily enjoyable e. optional f. enjoyable and important g. enjoyable but not particularly important h. so much a part of routine that they are practically unnoticed	*Consider:* other categories, besides those listed, that would be helpful in establishing and ordering the importance of various activities to Mrs. B
List all the activities in the order of priority that you consider to be essential if Mrs. B is to continue with a way of living that would be socioculturally	*(Interpretation of data)* *Consider:* Mrs. B's thoughts and feelings about your list, and

Initial Assessment	Notes
acceptable and personally satisfying	therefore possible modifications
2. From the assessment of Mrs. B's motor, sensory, intellectual, and integrative functioning, list:	
a. the *difficulties* she is likely to encounter in the performance of each activity listed. (Separate those unaffected, those able to be performed with adaptations or modifications, and those unable to be performed.)	*Consider:* slow, laborious movements generally; upper limb motions linked in synergies; spasticity; frail physical condition; slight aphasia; depression; neglect of upper limb; home environment (need more information on physical layout and possible architectural barriers), including relatively long solitary periods at home
b. the *strengths* she has that will enable her to overcome or compensate for these difficulties	*Consider:* attitudes, motivation, residual physical capacities, positive aspects of home and community environment, interpersonal relationships, interests, problem-solving skills
c. the new skills (or methods) she might have to acquire to help her cope with, or compensate for, these difficulties	*Consider:* expansion of environment and interests; acquisition of compensatory skills, e.g., one-handed activities by means of improved dexterity on unaffected side; learning of new methods, e.g., different organization of field of action, such as objects placed and stored within easy reach; use of adaptive equipment

Initial Assessment	*Notes*
3. List the additional information (and the sources of this information) essential for the treatment plan	*Consider:* prognosis {expected duration of stay at center — physician} Coordination of scheduling, and integration of program goals {program for walking, managing steps, position of upper limb while doing these activities — physical therapist; prognosis for aphasia and reading and writing problems, if any — speech therapist}

Planning	*Notes*
1. List the overall goals of occupational therapy for Mrs. B in the light of Mrs. B's activities configuration, difficulties, and strengths	State goals in relation to the *behaviors* that will indicate that Mrs. B has attained maximal activities health, e.g., pride in keeping home neat and clean, which is a pointer to activities health and relates to ability to (fill in what is appropriate): . . . . . Similarly, maintaining church activities relates to ability to (fill in what is appropriate): . . . . .
2. List the attainable steps (short-term goals) by which the ultimate goals can be reached. List these steps in order of priority, indicating expected time for attainment of each.	*Consider:* constraints of time, the clinical situation, and the home environment *Notes:* this particular clinical setting has two separate rooms — one for general activities and the

Planning	Notes
	other set up for homemaking; daily half-hour periods (Monday to Friday) are available
3. Adapt or modify activities in their field of action when necessary: a. environments b. objects c. people	*Consider:* special equipment to facilitate one-handed activities using affected side as assist, e.g., one-handed jar-openers; stabilizers for bowls, pots, and pans; organization of supplies in the most accessible way. *Do not* use special equipment in any instance if Mrs. B can manage without it in comfort and safety. *Also consider:* incorporation of affected upper limb in symmetrical, bilateral movements to prevent neglect of affected limb and to reeducate patterns of movement — use of adapted equipment (example in Fig. 8-1). *Consider:* other people to be introduced into Mrs. B's program: groups in clinic? her husband? 16-year-old friend? contacts from church?
4. Consider precautions to be taken	Minimize neglect of upper limb — give constant encouragement to keep limb in view during activity. Watch for associated reactions in affected limb (increase of spasticity) with forceful movements of unaffected limb. *Consider:* reflex inhibiting positions while one-sided activities

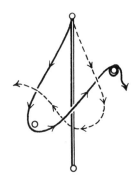

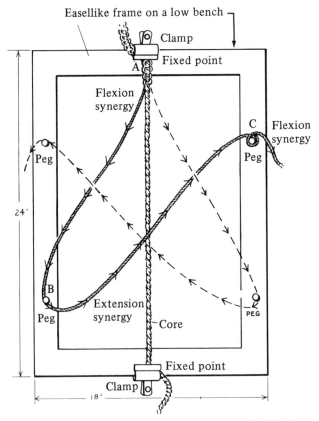

Figure 8-1. Macramé adapted as a therapeutic activity for Mrs. B, a patient with right hemiplegia.

Planning	Notes
	are being carried out (see Bobath [7]).
	Watch for environmental objects or situations that have become hazards because of unilateral neglect, loss of kinesthetic awareness in elbow and shoulder, slowness of motions, e.g., hot stove, projections on which affected limb can catch, disturbance of body balance while reaching over stove or kitchen sink. Do not allow overexertion.
	Remember fatigue — physical condition plus depression.
	Grade activity in terms of duration and difficulty.
	Watch for correct positioning of head, neck, trunk, and upper and lower limbs in all activities.
5. Draw up a weekly schedule blank, and fill in timetable for each anticipated step in the program — periods per day, days per week	Morning and afternoon sessions are available; duration of stay depends on third-party payments, but extension can be obtained if patient's condition warrants it; additional environments available
6. Select activities that will facilitate attainment of goals	are a library, unit dayroom, gift shop, cafeteria, and long, seldom-frequented corridors in a research wing — all within the center; outside are busy streets and shops.
Check: — Meaning and relevance	Some suggestions for now and later as Mrs. B progresses: simple cooking, dishwashing, bedmaking,

Planning	*Notes*
	and other household maintenance tasks, especially *dusting* and *polishing* (work out why); knotting macramé straps and shoulder sling for book holder on a specially adapted frame, ensuring that Mrs. B incorporates movement patterns that she has to make each knot (see Fig. 8-1); if macramé is unfamiliar to you, consult instruction book or leaflet; helping in library — e.g., sorting books and stacking from wheeled cart; presenting a story to a group of children, including selecting, summarizing, writing (or maybe typing) notes, and presenting. Refer back to activities configuration and activities history.
— Fulfilling conditions for arousing and harnessing will to learn	Read Chapter 4, pp. 35–43
— Organization in systematic way based on a rationale that takes into consideration physical and psychosocial problems.	The physical assessment was based to some degree on Brunnstrom's [11] system. How does this fit in as a treatment approach? (Use Appendix 4 as a guide.)
7. Organize activities in a regular schedule (fill in schedule blank) allowing for gradual increase in time, difficulty, and variety of activity	

Implementation

Without an actual patient who responds and reacts, Mrs. B's program from here on becomes purely hypothetical. There are, however, ways to practice the general principles of implementation. Some are presented here. Others will most certainly occur to you.

1. Set up the macramé project as depicted in Figure 8-1. Explain its purpose to an individual who is playing the role of the patient (a fellow student, colleague, or captive friend). Teach the activity to the patient, making sure you have broken it down into manageable steps. At the end of the session (half an hour, as in the clinic), mark progress and prepare "patient" for the next step.

    Try to observe a patient (or better still, patients) whose physical functioning approximates that of Mrs. B. How do you think they could cope with the activity as you taught it to your substitute patient? If you have the chance, try it out with a patient. Many patients, like Mrs. B, are intrigued and stimulated by taking part in a new project; others may find the situation too threatening.

    Note. Watch positioning throughout the activity and check pacing. Check that the "patient" has mastered what you have taught.
2. Set up any other activity in a field of action that you have included in your plan for Mrs. B. Test it out with a substitute patient or, if you can do so appropriately, with a real patient.
3. Consider the following questions, which materially affect implementation:
    a. How would you introduce the program and the very first activity to Mrs. B? (Practice different approaches. Exchange ideas with fellow students or your supervisor or colleagues.)
    b. What signal behaviors would tell you that it is an appropriate time to introduce changes in the program?
    c. What kind of a contract for interaction would you set up with Mrs. B, bearing in mind her difficulties, strengths, and striving toward independence? How would you specifically carry out this contract in terms of the goals that have been set and the timetable you have drawn up?

Termination

Assuming that Mrs. B, within two weeks of her announced discharge date, has in the three and a half months of her stay attained all but the final steps that you have determined as important:

1. Write a discharge plan that follows the principles set out in Chapter 7, pp. 71–74.
2. Evaluate her total program. What would you have added, omitted, changed? Why?

9. Case 2. P

P is 6 years and 9 months old. He is somewhat shorter than average, thin, and wiry, with a mop of red-gold curls and bright blue eyes. He is currently enrolled in a first-grade program at a public school. As part of his program at school, he attends a special physical education session once a week for children with learning disabilities, is enrolled in a program that deals with auditory discrimination for assistance with spelling, and is in a special reading class. He has been referred to occupational therapy because of a series of problems noted by his teachers.

General Background and Family Style of Living

In addition to eight months of first grade, P's formal educational program has included nine months of a half-day kindergarten program and 12 months of a daily preschool program. The family moved into the present school district at the beginning of the current school year. They reside in a three-bedroom apartment in a complex that has indoor and outdoor recreational facilities for children. P is the oldest child and has a room of his own. His two younger siblings, both girls, are 4 years and 18 months old, respectively. He does not have any close friends with whom to play, although there are many children available at the complex.

The father's work in sales requires him to travel during the week, but he is home for weekends. The mother works part-time as a clerical helper in an office and is away from home during the school hours. The two younger children attend a day care center. The mother drives P and his sisters to and from school or the day care center.

Functional History

P's mother gives the following history. P has difficulties in learning to read, print, and spell. His performance in mathematics and science is outstanding. During school hours he cannot sit still, talks aloud frequently, does not follow simple school rules, and cries easily. He is apparently having difficulties with his peer group and is also difficult for the teachers to handle. On the playground P does not join in group activities. He will "strike out" at other children and seems very "clumsy" in playground activities. P hates school because the children tease him about his clumsiness and call him "Dum-dum." The teachers requested that P be seen by a pediatrician to rule out physical causes for his school difficulties and to obtain advice about the proper kind of approach to P. Both the kindergarten and preschool teachers had reported and discussed difficulties similar to those that P now has at school.

School Reports

The teachers report that P has been tested by the school psychologist and a speech pathologist. Tests administered by the school during the past few months have included the Wechsler Intelligence Scale for Children (WISC), the Bender-Gestalt Test, the Illinois Test of Psycholinguistic Abilities (ITPA), and the Frostig Developmental Test of Visual Perception. Results indicate that P has above-average intellectual ability, the verbal subtests of the WISC being superior to the performance subtests. The Bender-Gestalt Test indicated possible organic causes for P's behavior and apparent visual-motor difficulties. There is evidence of both auditory and visual perceptual problems, relating to auditory discrimination and sequencing, visual form constancy, and figure-ground discrimination. Auditory and visual memory appears adequate. The specifics of these reports are not available, because P's father refused to sign a release, demanding that no results appear as part of P's school records.

The teachers confirmed the description of P's behavior given by the mother, saying that she is most cooperative in every way and tries to carry out their suggestions in the home. They feel that the current programs are helping P, and that it would be helpful for him to repeat first grade next year. P has missed many days of school because of frequent falls, upper respiratory infections (URIs), and stomach problems. During school he falls frequently and has to visit the school nurse for minor care at least twice a week.

Pediatrician's Report

The pediatrician reports that he has seen P on three occasions. The last visit was requested by the teachers because of P's school problems. P has a history of frequent URIs, allergies, the usual childhood diseases, and two arm fractures. His height, weight, and head circumference are within normal limits. Neurological screening indicates some soft neurological signs — P cannot stand on one foot, is unable to hop or skip, and has difficulty with fast alternating movements of his upper extremities. There is a very mild intention tremor in the fingers, and muscles appear to be slightly hypotonic. P has had examinations of both hearing and vision within the past six months. No complications were noted. No medication was prescribed. P has been given a diet that eliminates all food additives, artificial coloring, and white sugar.

Parental Attitudes

P's mother is most cooperative, giving whatever information is requested, because she is so relieved that P is getting help and that so many people are showing an interest in him. She diligently carries through programs and regimens recommended and tries not to let her irritation with P or frustration at being unable to get through to him at times force her into punitive action.

She receives very little support from her husband, who, she feels, laughs at her when she tries to approach the subject of P's difficulties. P's father refused to participate in a conference with the occupational therapist, even though a weekend time for meeting was suggested, and similarly refused to enter into a discussion by telephone. He denies that there is a problem, saying that P's mother and the teachers are making matters worse by interfering. He is certain that P will "grow out of" his clumsiness and inability to spell and read, just as he himself did. The root of the matter, he feels, is that the schools do not enforce discipline, and that the reason the teachers cannot control P is that "he is too smart for them." He plans to send P to a military prep school when the boy is 10 years old.

Occupational Therapy Assessment

The occupational therapy evaluation reveals sensory-motor integrative difficulties, which contribute to P's learning and behavior problems.

Southern California Sensory Integration Tests
The results of P's performance range from a standard score of +0.1 to a
-2.5. The scores on the subtests are given in Table 9-1.

Table 9-1. Subtest Scores

Manual form perception	+0.1	Localization of tactile stimuli	-1.3
Rt.-lt. discrimination	+0.0	Standing balance – eyes closed	-2.5
Finger identification	-2.3	Standing balance – eyes open	-1.7
Position in space	-1.7	Crossing midline of body	-2.0
Double tactile stimuli	-1.2	Figure-ground perception	-0.0
Kinesthesia	-1.4	Bilateral motor coordination	-2.4
Motor accuracy – rt.	-2.3		
Motor accuracy – lt.	-2.5	CMLX rt.	-1.8
		CMLX lt.	-0.8
Space visualization	-1.9		

*Functional Assessment (from Observation and
Activities Performance)*
P has immature equilibrium reactions with poor midline stability. His
postural control is influenced by primitive righting reactions. Under
stress or when fatigued, P cannot differentiate head and trunk movements, so when he turns his head the entire trunk turns with it, affecting performance of the tasks to which he is attending.

Prehension patterns are immature. He begins an activity with full prehension but as he fatigues he regresses to pincer or total grasp. He has
an unusually tight grip. He seems to prefer to use his left hand but will
switch during an activity.

As he works at desk activities he loses control of posture and needs
external props to maintain an erect sitting position. He has difficulty
using scissors and substitutes for normal grasp with an immature palmar
grasp and forearm pronation. He tends to abduct and hyperextend his

fingers when releasing objects held in his hand. P shows signs of tactile defensiveness. He is easily distracted, is in constant motion, and appears to be "driven" to move without apparent purpose.

P is motivated to participate in the occupational therapy activities and seems pleased with whatever he accomplishes. He shows interest in the younger children around him. He seems to have some understanding of his problem. Once he told the therapist that he could not think about how to print letters and learn what they looked like because "my mind just won't let me do two things at a time."

Developmental and Play History (Obtained from Mother and P's Baby Book)

Infancy

P had UR infections and some wheezing; he was allergic to milk and was put on a soybean formula diet. Infant feeding time was difficult — it was hard for P to suck from the nipple of his bottle and his mother had to cut larger holes for him to manage. P was a "fussy" baby, who never seemed to enjoy being held or rocked. He spent most of his first six months in his infant seat or on his back in the crib or on the floor. He liked watching mobiles, sucking on toys, or being talked or sung to. He would cry when placed on the floor on his tummy to play. He rolled over by himself at six months but never seemed to roll toward objects or for other specific purposes. He sat alone at seven months, crawled at nine months, and took his first steps at 15 months. The mother does not remember when he stood alone. He continued to walk and run on the tips of his toes until he was 5 years old.

Toddler Stage

P's father liked to "roughhouse" with him, but the child seemed quite frightened and started to scream, particularly when he was tossed in the air. P enjoyed playing with large wooden blocks, cars, and trucks for short periods. Play usually ended with P becoming frustrated because he could not get the blocks or cars to do what he wanted. His favorite activities were playing in the sandbox and with boats in the bathtub. When P was successful with an activity, his attention was "endless."

Motor Skills

P rode a "kiddy car" when he was 2 but was unable to ride a tricycle until he was 3 1/2 years old. His father made attempts to play catch with P, but the game usually ended in frustration for both. P accomplished climbing stairs at 4, after a great deal of difficulty, and climbed with alternating steps at 6. He still needs to use a handrail when descending.

P seldom engaged in activities requiring fine motor skills. He refused to finger-paint, scribbled aimlessly with crayons, and still has difficulty handling crayons and pencils. He began to use scissors for cutting paper at 4 but is still unable to use them proficiently.

Self-Care

P fed himself finger foods at 12 months and handled a training cup and a spoon at approximately 15 months. He still is a "messy" eater and his poor table manners irritate his parents. They refuse to take him out to eat in public because he constantly spills food and drink.

P started to undress himself at age 3, and dress at 4. His biggest problem was differentiating top from bottom and inside from outside. He still buttons his shirts in a careless manner (third buttonhole matching first button). He can tie his shoes, slowly and with difficulty. He is encouraged to take care of his own dressing, but his mother reports that she usually ends up doing the task for him on school mornings, rather than trying to "push him along."

Peer Relationships and General Activity

At home P prefers to stay indoors and watch TV. While he is watching he frequently jumps from chair to chair, attempts to turn somersaults, and jumps up and down. At times he is so active that his mother makes him go to his room and get control of himself.

She often insists that he go outside to play, but within ten minutes he comes in crying, saying that "the kids hit me." Mother reports that P has never been able to play with other children without getting into fights. She has tried a variety of methods to improve the situation, from coaxing to forcing, but nothing seems to work.

Because of P's difficulties with peer relationships, the mother has sought out a variety of youth programs at the local YMCA. P starts out pleased, but after three or four tries he wants to stop. Swimming has been the most successful activity. He is proud that he can jump off the diving board and swim to the edge of the pool. P's two greatest wishes are to be able to ride his bicycle without training wheels, and to be able to bat a baseball when he plays with his father.

The Occupational Therapy Program
1. Follow the guidelines given for Mrs. B, adapting them to P's particular situation.
2. Compare and contrast the total programs for Mrs. B and P.

Consider:
1. The implications of the Southern California Sensory Integration Tests results — interpretation of data for program planning; linkage to function or dysfunction; explanation in terms parents and teachers can comprehend and act upon
2. The relationship of these results to the functional assessment
3. The theoretical approach/approaches to be used as a rationale for systematic organization of activities
4. The family situation
5. P's activities configuration
6. P's chronological age and developmental level
7. P's difficulties and strengths
8. P's needs and wants

Notes
The occupational therapist to whom P has been referred has a private practice in a clinic located close to P's school.

10. Case 3. Mr. S

Mr. S is a 35-year-old baker who was admitted to the hospital two weeks ago, after attacking his employer with a kitchen knife. The employer, Mr. V, was not hurt, but he claims that Mr. S threatened him with violence on several occasions, shouting, "Why are you making me put poison in the bread?"

General Appearance and Behavior
Mr. S walked into the occupational therapy department with a shuffling gait, head down. He is tall and very thin, with sunken cheeks accentuated by a dark stubble. His clothes are rumpled and his thick dark hair, which he wears rather long, is disheveled. His shoes are cracked and unpolished, and the loosely tied laces trail along the ground. Although it is chilly, he wears no socks and his open-necked shirt, with a top button missing, leaves his neck and upper chest exposed. His baggy sweater is stained. He smokes incessantly, and his fingers are stained with nicotine. His nails are bitten, though quite clean. In conversation he started by mumbling and avoided eye contact, but he became more relaxed and spoke more clearly as the session proceeded. He was at all times able to give coherent replies to questions and to initiate a few conversational gambits of his own. He concentrated hard on the questionnaires and forms he was asked to fill in and completed them rapidly.

Background Information (from Intake Notes)

Family History
Mr. S was born in Greece but came to America with his parents when he was 3 years old. His father died of leukemia when he was 5. The father, 35 at the time of his death, had worked as a short-order cook in an uncle's restaurant, and his mother did "a little bit of dressmaking" for neighbors and relatives. Relatives had to help the struggling widow

and her young child for three years. She refused to live with the uncle and his children, claiming she had too much pride to live on the charity of her in-law family, but she had to accept their offers of financial help, which she regarded as a loan. Mr. S remembers her "always dressed in black, never a smile, never a soft word, old before her time."

The mother remarried when Mr. S was 8. Mr. S's stepfather was an American of Italian-Greek parentage. A widower, 25 years older than his wife, with grown-up children from his first marriage, he adopted Mr. S, who took his stepfather's second name. According to Mr. S, he was "a kind man, always smiling, always wanting to be a nice guy, gave me a lot of presents, money – lots of things."

Mr. S says he had a happy time at home until he was 17, when his stepfather "did a terrible thing." Mr. S was unable to discuss this further, but relatives subsequently revealed that the stepfather had been convicted of embezzlement and sentenced to an eight-year prison term; he died of a heart attack a year later.

At the time of the "terrible thing," his mother went into a deep depression and attempted suicide. She was hospitalized in a state institution for about three months, given shock treatment, and sent home; there she "mooned around, hardly ever speaking, carried out her jobs at home all right, but did nothing else except go to church and cry." After her return from the hospital, Mr. S moved with his mother to a self-contained part of a house owned by his uncle. All his father's relatives were very helpful at this stage. On the other hand, the stepfather's family withdrew completely after the "disgrace," and Mr. S has had no further contact with them since.

These troubles affected Mr. S's schoolwork. He had been a hardworking student with average grades and was set on earning his high school diploma, despite the fact that he disliked school. However, he left school in the twelfth grade, having stayed away from classes on a number of occasions. He claimed that he could not concentrate, and anyway had to go out and get work, because the stepfather had left them no money. Through the good offices of his uncle he was apprenticed as a baker to Mr. V, for whom he has worked ever since.

When Mr. S was 22 his mother made a second attempt at suicide, taking an overdose of sleeping pills. She was in a coma for four months before she died. He continued to live at his uncle's house for three years; then he married, against the advice of his relatives, a "no-good" woman of 28. She had a 7-year-old son by a previous marriage that had ended in divorce after her husband, an alcoholic, had severely beaten her and the child. Apparently she had been "keeping company" with another man at the time. According to the relatives, she was a good-looking blonde who liked "high living."

The newly married couple moved into an apartment in a nice neighborhood, and Mr. S had it "fixed up good." The wife started frequenting bars and "picking up" men early in the marriage. Their quarrels became frequent and violent, to the extent that the neighbors had to call the police on several occasions. Eventually, after a little more than a year, the wife disappeared, taking a large sum of money with her but leaving the child with Mr. S. He was "so disgusted" that he had the child put in a foster home − "I never did like that kid − sniveling, lying little _____!" He obtained a divorce five years after his wife left.

Mr. S moved back to the uncle's house when his wife left, and has lived there ever since.

Medical History

Mr. S had the usual childhood illnesses, mumps at 7, measles at 5, and occasional colds and sore throats. He now looks undernourished; he weighs 140 pounds and is 5 feet 11 inches tall. A thorough medical check-up, including neurological tests, shows no abnormalities. Mr. S says he is "strong as a horse," has never missed a day's work through illness, and has always eaten and slept well except for the past eight months, when he has had "terrible nightmares." His relatives urged him to get help when they discovered his drinking problem, but he says no doctor has the power to stop "them" (the evil ones). By the time Mr. S was admitted because of the attack on Mr. V, he was quite calm and rational and there have been no signs of recurrence of violent behavior. He is receiving no medication, and has made no mention of or indicated in other ways his need for alcohol.

General Style of Living

Interviews with Mr. S, his relatives, and Mr. V by occupational therapist and social worker. Mr. S lives in a large, comfortable three-story house owned by an uncle in a lower-middle-class neighborhood. He occupies a suite on the second floor, which consists of a large bed-sitting room and bathroom, comfortably furnished. He takes his meals — evening meal only, six days a week — with the family. Besides uncle, a hale and hearty 76, and aunt age 69 ("a wonderful cook and housewife"), two married cousins and their wives — all in the family restaurant business — occupy portions of the house divided into separate duplex apartments with their children — a total of three boys and two girls, ranging in age from 4 to 16. Two other of the uncle's grandchildren are away at college.

The extended family has strong bonds and everyone is very "emotional" and vociferous. All talk loudly and enthusiastically, and they "fight and love with gusto." Mr. S, though never overtalkative, was one of them before "his troubles." After that, he became morose and monosyllabic, although until his "breakdown" he showed his attachment to the family by a number of touching gestures — remembering birthdays with gifts of beautifully decorated cakes, offering to babysit for the little ones, mending a broken toy or household appliance, helping with household chores.

Mr. S gets up at 4:30 A.M. six days a week and walks to work one mile from home. He starts work at 5:30, takes a quick breakfast — although he is allowed a 45-minute break when the first batches of rolls and Danish pastries are ready for the oven — and then works until 1:30. Before his breakdown he used to stroll to a nearby coffee shop for lunch, sit in the park reading a newspaper left lying around or "just watching," or play a game of boccie (an Italian version of bowling) with a group of old-timers. In bad weather he would go to the local bar, linger over a drink, and watch TV. He returns from his lunch break at 3:00 and works until 5:00, preparing the dough for the early morning baking, except on Saturdays, when he finishes work for the day at about 2:00.

About eight months ago he started going straight to the bar every day during his afternoon break, downing "quite a few drinks" before going back to work. Neither his punctuality nor the quality of his work seemed to suffer.

Mr. V says that Mr. S is a "fantastic" worker, very diligent and conscientious to the point where he refuses to take time off due to him. He is careful and "artistic" — he decorates all the cakes, designing "from his head" as he goes along. The bakery has an excellent reputation and is always crowded with customers. Mr. V manages the tiny shop, while he lets Mr. S be "king" in the kitchen, lording it over the two helpers. This has been the only source of friction in the 15 years Mr. S has been a master baker. He bullies his helpers, drives them hard, and complains all the time that the new generation does not know what hard work and quality mean. In the last four or five months Mr. S has become even more suspicious, bad-tempered, and demanding, and he has leveled accusations of poisoning attempts at Mr. V three or four times. Nothing specific seemed to precipitate the outbursts of shouting, obscene language, threats, and finally the physical assault directed at Mr. V. Mr. S says Mr. V has been a fair and good boss, but the "devils" have got hold of Mr. V and must be removed.

After work Mr. S, until recently, took the bus home, went up to his room, and took a nap until dinner time, which is punctually at 7:00. Generally the two or three adults working in the restaurant are absent from the family meal. Mr. S participated very little in conversation at the table. He went back to his room immediately after dinner, watched TV, did a few chores like sewing on buttons, or played solitaire, and went to bed at ten o'clock. Occasionally he babysat, joined the children in a game of Monopoly, or helped them with crafts projects.

On Sundays the whole family gathers for an elaborate meal at noon that goes on for several hours. Mr. S, until his strange behavior took over, always joined the family and sat in the living room afterward reading the newspapers, mainly the sports and travel sections. He was without fail invited to family outings and celebrations but declined unless the gatherings took place at home. At these he was usually to be found playing cards with a group of men he had known for years. Mr. S says he at one time enjoyed going down to the "club" (an informal gathering of men from the neighborhood in one of the old-fashioned food store-cum-cafés that are rarely found nowadays) to play cards, especially pinochle, drink wine or beer, and chat. For the rest of the Sunday, he used to take a walk, watch TV, or help his uncle with a few maintenance chores around the house. For supper he would fix a sandwich and take it up to his room.

Since his breakdown he has gone up to his room after work and has refused to take evening meals with the family. His food, brought on a tray, is eaten very sparingly, but he drinks all evening until he falls asleep. On Sundays, until a few weeks before his attack on Mr. V, he made an effort to join the family at the noon meal, interacted with them to some extent as before, but went upstairs to his solitary drinking in the late afternoon.

According to his aunt, Mr. S used to make his bed before going to work, and leave his room clean and tidy. He dressed neatly and "quite elegantly" and was very particular to keep his hands clean. He always smoked heavily, but aired his room and cleaned out the ashtrays before leaving for work. He did his own cleaning and mending of clothes. But a few months ago he began to look slovenly. He stopped going to the barber regularly every two weeks for a trim, and his clothes became creased and dirty. Instead of neatly making his bed, he pulled the cover over the tumbled bedclothes; he left his room messy, clothes tossed on chairs, ashtrays filled with cigarette butts, a dirty glass on the table. However, he always hid the empty bottles after his drinking bouts.

Activities History (Occupational Therapy)

Mr. S filled in a questionnaire designed to provide information about his activities history and also filled in a checklist for an interest inventory. The information obtained was discussed with Mr. S at a subsequent interview. He left the answers blank for all questions that dealt with hopes and aspirations. For many of the questions dealing with the interpersonal relationships involved in activities, he wrote: "It's a lot of _____" or "More _____" or "Who cares?" The following is a summary of the information obtained from the questions he completed, the checklist he filled in, and the interview.

Mr. S was an average student at public school, which he attended until he was 9 years old. He worked hard and passed all his subjects. He had no favorites but did well in mathematics and drawing. His worst subject was English. At school he felt "different," because all the other children had spending money and wore nice clothes. His mother considered pocket money an extravagance and saw no reason why he should not wear hand-me-downs from his cousins, which she remodeled for him. He cannot remember any teachers whom he particularly liked. He had one or two friends from class with whom he played a variety of ball games in the street after school.

His life changed in a number of ways when his mother remarried. He was sent to a parochial school with a fine reputation, but he disliked the "uppishness" of most of the teachers and the emphasis on academic excellence. By working very hard he just managed to attain passing grades. The art teacher was the only one Mr. S remembers with warmth. This was the person who encouraged Mr. S to go on to get his high school diploma and continue with his drawing and design, the one subject at which he excelled. Mr. S disliked any group activities and got into trouble several times for cutting gym classes and team sports. Yet he enjoyed physical activity — walking, running, bicycling — that he could do on his own. His stepfather lavished gifts on him — books, records, expensive construction kits, musical instruments ("I've got no feel for music"), games, sports equipment, clothes. He tired very quickly of these objects, and he still felt "different" at school, despite the fact that he now had the right clothes and ample pocket money.

The childhood objects Mr. S considered important and for which he felt affection were a model train set he received from his uncle for Christmas when he was 7 years old, a number of coloring books, and modeling clay, which he hoarded for a long time. The only object given to him by his stepfather, which he still cherishes, and, in fact, has mounted on the wall of his room, is a fishing rod. His stepfather used to take him fishing at dawn on Sundays. His mother was too "cheap" to give him presents, even when her financial situation improved.

The objects that are important to Mr. S now are his TV set, playing cards, his cake-decorating tools, and his baker's hat. His list of hobbies and interests encompasses work — especially cake-decorating and shaping rolls and cakes; watching TV; walking; fixing things — broken toys, toasters, and so on; and playing cards, especially solitaire.

Asked how he would sum up his general style of living before he "got sick," he said that he had been pretty comfortable — no money problems, no women problems, no work problems except for those fresh kids — before people (not specified) started bugging him with their wrongdoing. He had always lived a clean, decent life and "they" were out to spoil his record. Those "devils" all around were at work to make something terrible happen. To the question about what he most wanted to do with his life, he replied, without any change of emotional tone; "To be left alone."

The Occupational Therapy Program

1. Follow the guidelines given for Mrs. B, adapting them to Mr. S's particular situation.
2. You will note that no interpretations have been made of Mr. S's behavior. Discuss, preferably with a group, the implications of Mr. S's behavior from several different theoretical viewpoints that you are familiar with. This will help you select a theoretical rationale that will provide the basis for a systematic approach to Mr. S's occupational therapy program.
3. Compare and contrast the three occupational therapy programs.

Consider:

Mr. S's present behavior, immediate past behavior, and general patterns of acting, reacting, and interacting

Mr. S's activities configuration

Mr. S's family dynamics and their relationship to his behavior with Mr. V and the two helpers at work

The contract for interaction to be set up between the occupational therapist and Mr. S

Notes

Mr. S has been admitted to a hospital that has inpatient, outpatient, day-care, and a number of satellite community programs. He is now in an observation unit of the inpatient section, sharing a room with a man of his own age. The general philosophy of the hospital encompasses a commitment to the therapeutic community (see reference to Maxwell Jones in Suggested Readings). Occupational therapy is integrated into an interdisciplinary activities program that includes music therapy, recreational therapy, art therapy, and dance therapy. The activities center serves all sections of the hospital and is large and well-equipped. The hospital stands in large, wooded grounds in the community that it serves.

11. Brief Case Histories

B, Age 16

Referred to prevocational evaluation unit as outpatient. Lives at a home for disturbed boys, where he was sent after he appeared before a judge on charges of assaulting a teacher. Receives counseling daily. Home allows acting out and has very few rules for daily behavior. Has dropped out of school; was considered of below-average intelligence. Comes from a "decent" home — hard-working father, a watchmaker; mother at home with younger brother, age 7. Mother is very helpless and dependent on father. Has history of delinquent acts since 12 — stealing cars, passing drugs. Is short for his age, very good-looking; he affects an aggressive, don't-care manner. At initial assessment showed hostility, testing limits continually. Shows definite aptitude for drawing, which confirms school performance records. Contrary to school assessments, he appears very intelligent — has read lives of artists, taught himself anatomy for sketching from manuals, and remembers and identifies names of muscles. Knows he is unable to get on with authorities; finds teachers "stupid" and uncaring. Would like to be a famous artist but does not see why he has to go to school for it — after all, Da Vinci didn't!

N, Age 7 1/2

Referred for occupational therapy after hospitalization for resection of recurrent cerebellar astrocytoma, complicated by hydrocephalus requiring shunting. N is youngest of three daughters of Pakistani family who lived in the United States until N was 4 1/2. They moved back to Pakistan, where N started school at age 6. Initial tumor resection was done at 2 1/2 years without complications. Mother describes normal motor, adaptive, and language development so far. History indicates excellent school performance (second grade) and well- adjusted social interaction. A major focus of her present play repertoire includes organization of a "secret society" of female peers. Postsurgical physical assessment shows fluctuating muscle tone from mild hypotonicity to moderate hypertonicity. All movements and posture are dominated by reflex reactions, particularly the asymmetrical tonic neck reflex. Voluntary motions are limited to head-raising in prone position, rolling with minimal assistance, and gross arm movement on the right. Feeding is complicated by rooting and biting reflexes, left facial spasticity, and right facial flaccidity. Mother is currently feeding her with a syringe. N is unable to produce voluntary vocalization. It is mother's impression that N understands what is said to her. Expressive aphasia is being considered.

Miss F, Age 82

Miss F looks younger and sprightlier than 82. Worked all her life as writer/editor in publications related to entertainment. In later years, lifelong hobby of painting became primary occupation, with active painting, selling, and exhibiting. Lived with sister, who also never married, also is a career woman, also young-looking, but reportedly not as successful as patient. Both are "sort of" Christian Scientists.

Hospitalized for a myocardial infarct (has a history of cardiac problems) with a residual hemiplegia and expressive aphasia. Because of advanced age, medical history, and severe expressive aphasia, she was not considered a good rehabilitation candidate and indeed was rushed out of the hospital in three weeks. She was referred to Home Care Service and obtained a privately paid full-time attendant. Home care includes social service, PT, OT, and speech therapy. Physical status: almost nonexistent speech (receptivity intact), severe spasticity on right side, no sitting or standing balance, facial paralysis.

Complications: sister's oversolicitousness – she insists attendant do everything for patient, waits unrealistically for the day patient will be "all better" – and patient's inability to convey any disagreement with her sister because of her aphasia.

L, Age 33

Has been in institutions for the mentally retarded since the age of 16. Lived with grandmother before that; mother abandoned him, father unknown. When grandmother died, was sent to state institution, where he remained until three months ago, when institution was closed because of public outcry. He was transferred to another state facility, which has a much better reputation. At the time he was referred to occupational therapy, he was confined to a cottage because of his repulsive personal habits. Although his personal hygiene and dressing are attended to by the nursing staff, he is unkempt, clothes unbuttoned and food-stained. He eats "like an animal," wolfing his food in great chunks, allowing it to dribble down his face and clothes, unable to use knife and fork, and making loud, repellent noises when he drinks. He takes his meals alone because the residents refuse to have him around while they are eating. His greatest wish is to have coffee with the others in the dining room.

AL, Age 27

Married, with daughter age 3. Has diagnosis of multiple sclerosis. Symptoms began five years ago. Lives in two-bedroom apartment in elevator building with husband and child. Mother lives nearby and appears to be a strong family figure, having brought up seven children without a father. AL was studying part-time for a social work degree but left on account of illness after 3 1/2 years. She resigned from her job as part-time family counselor at a day care center one year ago. While she worked, her mother took care of the baby. The husband is director of a city community center. Both are involved in radical Black political groups.

Functional level: lives in a wheelchair, although she can ambulate short distances. Is independent in activities of daily living. Home responsibilities include meal preparation, house cleaning, caring for child. Husband seems to be removing himself from the picture.

Mr. G, Age 50

Warehouse guard. Has history of depressive episodes, during which he becomes agitated and fearful. Was hospitalized at 21 for several months and had shock treatments. Has now been admitted to a psychiatric ward because he has threatened suicide, refuses to go to work, cannot make himself get up in the mornings, paces back and forth when he is up, and blames himself for his wife's death two years ago. He lives with his only daughter and son-in-law. His three grandchildren do not get on with Mr. G — he claims they are "fresh" and inconsiderate, while they think he is an interfering bore, always telling them how good things were in his day. Mr. G was always a rather passive individual, leaving major decisions to his wife. His chief interests are watching TV and placing bets on horses.

J, Age 21

Sales assistant admitted to a psychiatric hospital with diagnosis of acute schizophrenia — withdrawn, confused, flat affect, psychomotor retardation. Put on medication and referred to occupational therapy a few days later. Was able to give history: lives with mother and a younger brother and sister in a city housing project, never had more than one or two friends, unable to socialize easily. Did not complete high school — school did not seem safe with assaults and muggings — although she received good grades. Found a job as a part-time helper in a department store at 17; was promoted to full-time gift wrapper at 18, because she was so neat and accurate. Has no hobbies or special interests but would like to "learn" some. Her occupational therapy activities evaluation revealed ability to follow directions (both written and oral) with facility, excellent manual skills, poor interpersonal skills, good concentration; flat affect throughout.

M, Age 9

Acute episode of juvenile rheumatoid arthritis, accompanied by depression, low frustration tolerance, decreased muscle strength (especially in proximal groups), and decreased sitting and standing tolerance. M wears a vertical spinal brace designed to maintain alignment and prevent pain associated with vertebral osteoporosis. Originally the brace was prescribed solely for ambulation, but M has become increasingly fearful of its removal and is reported to sleep with it on. The brace reinforces his rigid posture and hinders all flexion, preventing carrying out of manual tasks. He has been out of school for six months and has no appropriate peer contacts. M requires moderate assistance for transfer and total assistance for dressing and is independent only in self-feeding. His struggles to gain greater independence are hampered by his widowed mother's inconsistency — supporting independence within the home but resisting the push to regain normal school/play activity. Currently M spends all free time watching television and reading a little. He is interested in many craft activities, especially model car building, which he learned in the course of multiple hospitalizations.

Mr. D, Age 69

Admitted to a nursing home after a long hospitalization for a second coronary attack in the last 11 years. Lived alone in a room above the general store; there he helped with odd jobs, passed the time of day with the customers, to whom he was the town character, and kept a wary eye and ear open for intruders after hours. Has made a good physical recovery, despite the need to avoid too much exertion, but he is very lonely and depressed. His wife died 20 years ago, and one son, a merchant marine officer, has lived in Australia for many years. A daughter, an aspiring stage actress, visits him occasionally between marriages and acting engagements. Before his retirement because of illness at 59, Mr. D was a food inspector. His hobbies are gardening, collecting postcards from around the world, and reading adventure stories. He was also "quite a dancer" before he had his coronary attacks.

GD, Age 23

Was knocked over by a car that mounted the sidewalk. Suffered a head injury, resulting in ataxia, severe intention tremor in the right upper limb, loss of memory, and thickness of speech. GD comes from a family of high achievers. His father is a well-known businessman divorced from his mother, who is an ardent feminist and a very successful advertising executive. At the time of his accident, GD was a fourth-year student at a prestigious school of business administration. He was referred as an outpatient to the occupational therapy clinic six months after discharge from his initial hospitalization with the following problems: inability to concentrate, inability to write (because of intention tremor, unnoticeable until he begins a manual task), which provokes great anxiety about his ability to complete his studies; flashes of irritability and anger; fleeting lapses of consciousness; feeling unsteady on his feet. He has been going to typing classes in the hope of compensating for his inability to write and has been driving himself feverishly to get physically fit — practices the table of exercises given to him on discharge and does yoga and typing exercises at home. He is independent in all activities of daily living, including travel by subway. He manages steps, crowded trains, and streets but cannot run. Hobbies are reading — philosophy and modern novels — and table tennis. He likes going to parties and giving parties in the large home that he shares with his father.

ML, Age 13

Has systemic lupus erythematosus that has progressed to end-stage renal disease. Her present medical management includes renal dialysis three times per week.

Current status is characterized by functional psychosis, generalized muscle weakness, markedly decreased sitting and standing tolerance, and complete dependence in activities of daily living. She has immature behavior responses — screaming, crying, withdrawal from any attempts to assist her toward functioning. She is the second of four daughters born to a lower-class family. Parents are separated. She lives with mother. History, as related by mother, indicates adequate school performance, poor peer interaction at school, and leisure time spent in solitary creative tasks, e.g., crocheting, painting. Present physical appearance is marked by steroid side effects: loss of hair, cushingoid features, acne. She is, however, beginning to show some interest in grooming tasks such as hair styling and nail polishing.

C, Age 33

Quadriplegia at the level of C8, T1. Came from Puerto Rico 15 years ago and worked as a short-order cook for 12 years. In Puerto Rico his family was so poor that he had to leave school at 12 to go to work as a delivery boy. From the age of 8 he worked after school shining shoes and delivering newspapers. He was good at school; his best subject was mathematics, and he also excelled at sports — swimming, volleyball, and baseball. As an adult his favorite pastimes were movies, dancing and gambling. His spinal cord was severed six months ago by a bullet. Both lower extremities are flaccid; sitting balance is fair. He is right-dominant, but his left upper extremity is more functional than his right. C wants to use his right hand, which has a functional tenodesis grip. Functional motion strength in antigravity motions of the right upper extremity is G– in shoulder, elbow, and wrist. In the left upper extremity these motions are N. The left hand is F+ in metacarpophalangeal flexion and extension, and F– in thumb flexion and extension. Motivation is good, but C is depressed and angry. He has the promise of a fifth-floor studio apartment in an elevator building when he leaves the rehabilitation center. All his immediate family are in Puerto Rico.

P, Age 19

P has been a confirmed drug addict since the age of 12, when he started out as a pusher. Is an inpatient in a ward for young male addicts. Attends occupational therapy daily with a group of five wardmates. Is very verbal and uses his "erudite" vocabulary (having picked up a great deal of psychological jargon in his seven years in and out of hospitals and clinics) to avoid coming to grips with problems. A flashy dresser with a great deal of charm, he is obviously the leader of the group. He has a history of truancy, dropping out of school altogether at 13, and many delinquent acts, ranging from stealing from his foster mother to a number of muggings. He has managed to avoid prison by entering a drug rehabilitation program. Within the program he has achieved a degree of recognition for his aptitude for "fixing" things (from leaky faucets to crackling radios) and situations (for example, arranging for a last-minute replacement for a key player at a rock concert and negotiating for a pass to see a local movie).

Mrs. J, Age 54

Chronic rheumatoid arthritis affecting all joints, particularly severe in hands, wrists, and shoulders. She also has a cardiac problem. Is on a home health care program.

Mrs. J is dependent in all aspects of self-care. Ambulates with the aid of two canes.

Average day: Cousin reports that client sits in the chair in the living room and watches television. Male friend, F, returns home from work, and they both eat dinner. Cousin or F prepares meals and serves them.

Equipment: Double bed brought from client's bedroom on second floor and placed in the living room. A commode and canes are also used.

Client is on Medical Assistance.

Mrs. J's house is situated on a "stable" block on a street that divides a desolate factory area from a lower-class neighborhood. The inhabitants are Black and Puerto Rican.

The architectural barriers are numerous. To enter the house one walks up two cement steps to a three-foot-square landing, up nine ($1' \times 1'$) steps to another landing. There is a one-foot-wide cement structure that can be used for support while climbing the nine steps. The front door opens out, and one must climb up one more step to enter the porch.

The porch is littered with an old sofa and chairs, cardboard boxes, clothing, and broken lamps. There is one more step up to enter through glass doors into the living room. The interior of the house is orderly but dirty.

Mrs. J has one surviving daughter with two children. She will visit Mrs. J every other month or so but refuses to participate in caring for her. It is also reported that Mrs. J has few friends and few relatives who wish to help.

The supply of food is always limited to small quantities that could be bought at a nearby grocery store. Daily purchases of sausage, eggs, bread, tea, and beans are made — if there is someone available for the trip to the store. Mrs. J would rather smoke than eat.

The sink in the kitchen has no drain. Water can be drawn from the spigot, but refuse must be discarded in the bathroom on the second floor. Mrs. J says that she has no money to pay for this repair.

She wishes for only two things: to remain in her own home and to heat the house to 80 degrees. She has little concern for her well-being; she feels that she will eventually get the care that she needs. She is willing to wait for meals and care. The male friend does not seem interested in contributing to the expenses of running the house or in helping to care for her.

An Epilogue on the Art of Asking Questions

Research: "A search or investigation directed to the discovery of some fact by careful consideration of a subject; a course of critical or scientific inquiry." (*The Oxford English Dictionary*)

The preface to this book ended with a number of questions. Many other questions have been posed throughout the text. They ask why, how, and in which specific ways activities —which themselves need deeper scrutiny and investigation — are enlisted as therapeutic agents in the practice of occupational therapy. Further questioning will come with attempts to document the effects of this approach to practice on the individual, and to establish predictive criteria based on data related to activities functioning.

The areas for investigation are numerous and complex. To clarify the meaning and significance of *activities* necessitates the systematic collection of data about activities patterns and configurations in different sociocultural groups, interpretations and explanations of similarities and differences, and their importance to human functioning. The exploration of the process of *change* involves delving into learning mechanisms, motivation, human development and human relations, value systems, and human structure and function. The links between the hands and the brain are of particular significance to occupational therapy in this regard. Questions about change come tumbling: How does change in behavior from dysfunction to function take place? How is interest aroused and sustained? What are the similarities and differences between adult and child learning? What methods of instruction and interaction facilitate change? Which of these methods are most applicable to activities? Can these methods be applied generally? What methods best ensure integration of learning? How long does it take for change to take place? What are the optimum conditions for change to occur?

117

How is change defined and measured? What are the tools for measuring change?

The art of asking questions — the kinds of questions that lead to evaluation, reevaluation, and formulation and reformulation of theoretical propositions and clinical procedures — has to begin early. It is no accident that many of the assignments in this book include spurs to speculation and investigation. The contributions of students, clinicians, and educators who have developed the art of asking questions, who have sought out ways of answering them, and who have communicated the results of their endeavors are without doubt the basic building blocks for scientific research in occupational therapy. The development of the art of asking questions rests with a system of education that has as its core the manifesto propounded by Comenius (1592–1670) so many years ago:

"The Beginning and End of our Didactic will be: To seek and find a method by which the teachers teach less and the learners learn more."

Appendixes

Appendix 1. Activity Analysis Outline

The class will be divided into five groups of three people each. Each group is to select one activity of their own choice from the categories listed below:

1. Fine arts: e.g., sculpting, painting, music
2. Construction: e.g., woodworking, electronics assembly
3. Textiles: e.g., weaving, needlecraft
4. Games: e.g., checkers, golf
5. Domestic activities: e.g., cooking

Each group is to set up their own laboratory for purposes of exploring the activity and their individual and collective responses to it, and developing a detailed analysis based upon the attached outline. The resulting reports will be presented to the class the last week of the semester.

Outline
   I. *Definition and description* of the activity, including its stages and the apparatus, tools, and materials utilized
  II. *Manifest properties*
     A. Space occupied: Consider apparatus and procedures
     B. Time factors: Consider
        1. length of total experience
        2. length of each stage
        3. delays inherent in the process
        4. sequential ordering of stages linked with time
        5. rhythm and patterning of motions and processes
     C. Force: Requirements of the activity in terms of muscular tension and physical energy

   D. Interpersonal field:
   1. number of people involved
   2. nature of the transactions
      a. dependent
      b. independent
      c. cooperative
      d. collaborative
      e. competitive
   E. Sets: The variety of situations that characterize the process; e.g., a single process that is constant and predictable; shifting and varied processes or rules, or both
   F. Sensory input: color, texture, sound, odor, temperature (heat and cold)
   G. Sensory-motor integration: Opportunities for judgment of space, shape, texture, colors
   H. Kinetics: Motions involved in each stage of the process, e.g., starting position (sitting, standing, lying)
   1. changes in position
   2. main joints involved and their ranges
   3. muscle groups involved — kinds of muscle work done
   4. left/right comparison
   I. Cognitive skills required:
   1. Level of-thinking:
      a. sensory-motor, enactive, action
      b. concrete, iconic, imagery
      c. abstract, symbolic
   2. Memory: retention of information for steps, changes, procedures
   3. Levels of learning:
      a. reflexive
      b. cortical
      c. subcortical
   4. Degree of problem-solving and decision-making involved
   J. Cognitive-motor skills (manual dexterity) required
   K. Potential for self-expression and originality; creative thinking, planning, and implementation

L. Forms of communication:
  1. verbal
  2. nonverbal
  3. written
M. Opportunities for reality testing: representational or creative process; clearly established standards and techniques; extent to which structure or processes, or both, provide opportunity for agreement on the nature of reality; predictable results

III. *Acquired properties*
  A. Socioculturally determined attributes of objects, actions, and relationships based on:
    1. Notions of roles:
      a. age
      b. sex
      c. class
      d. status
        (1) occupational
        (2) educational
        (3) socioeconomic
    2. Impact of variations in religious and ethnic backgrounds
    3. Impact of historical social trends (past and present) and resulting attitudes toward activity
    4. Relevance of the activity or its parts to current concepts of work or recreation, or both
    5. Relevance to other activities of daily living, i.e., potential for integrated learning
  B. Personally determined attributes related to:
    1. Historical relevance: past experiences with the total activity, its stages, and its parts (objects, actions, interpersonal transactions); resulting attitudes, feelings, associations
    2. Symbolic meaning (collective and personal) of total activity, its stages, the process, its parts, and the end product
    3. Affective feeling states generated at different stages of the activity process
    4. The kinds of unconscious drives, needs, and feelings the activity process may potentially gratify. In what ways?

      5. New learning

      6. Old skills

      7. Ordering of old skills in new ways

      8. Idiosyncratic style of each individual

IV. *Adaptability*

    A. Environmental

    B. Interpersonal

    C. Apparatus

    D. To what degree do the inherent properties of the activity allow for realistic modification relative to the patient's needs and idiosyncratic style and to the patterns of activity in the real world?

Appendix 2. Activity Configuration Protocol

Client's Name   **MS** _____

Date _____

List below what you value most, the things *most important* to you now
and in the near future:

1. My kids — "I wouldn't want anything to happen to them. Don't
   know what I'd do if my parents didn't take care of them. I'm not a
   very good mother."
2. A happy family with a good father
3. Having a nice house and nice things
4. My religion — "Even though I'm not a very good Catholic."
5. My parents — "They're getting old. I don't want anything to happen
   to them."
6. Being loved by my husband — "But he probably doesn't want me
   back."
7. Looking nice — good figure, nice clothes. "If I hadn't got fat, my
   husband wouldn't have left me."
8. Having a good time and being happy
9. Dating — "I'd like to meet someone nice."

Educational History Interview

1. *What is your education?* (high school, college, other)
   High school (Catholic girls' school). Dropped out summer before
   senior year because of pregnancy.
2. *What were your major interests or areas of study?*
   Vocational major, secretarial course.
3. *What were your average grades? Were your grades better in some
   areas of study than in others?*

Usually Bs, honor roll a few times. Didn't do very well in math or science; did well in English and business courses.

4. *What did you like best about school?*
Secretarial, business, and English courses; drama club.

5. *What did you dislike about school?*
Not many friends; people jealous of my figure; sometimes made nasty remarks, usually comments not true.

6. *What did you think about your teachers? Did you have any favorites?*
Nuns very strict, but nice. Liked English teacher. She helped me write and said I was creative and sensitive. (Laugh.) Hasn't helped me much with my life (wistful expression).

7. *What were your spare time interests during your school years?*
Waitressing to save up for secretarial school; drama club, but couldn't go much because of working; movie magazines.

8. *What kind of things did you do with friends in school?*
Didn't really have many friends; sometimes hung out at pool hall or drugstore. Didn't date much — all the boys wanted was to "make out" or worse.

9. *What education did your parents have? Other members of your family?*
None, but worked very hard; wanted me to have an education. I really disappointed them.

10. *Do you have any future educational plans or interests?*
Maybe go to secretarial school or beauty school.

Other pertinent information (e.g., from school records, family, client formal testing):

Confirmation of educational history and concurrent social experiences given by parents in separate interview.

Summary and recommendations:

Explore possibility of MS taking high school equivalency exam.
Explore interests in secretarial or beauty school.

Work History Interview

Part I: Current or Most Recent Work Experience

1. *Where have you been working? How long?* Small manufacturing company (electronics) in same town I live in. Have been working there nine months; currently on sick leave. (My boss is getting divorced; it's my fault.)

2. *How do you get to work?* Take the bus to work. Sometimes a taxi if I oversleep.

3. *What kind of work have you been doing? What duties and skills are involved in your work? Have these been the same or have they changed since you've been working at this job?* Receptionist-clerk: answer telephone for personnel, bookkeeping, and secretarial offices; answer questions and direct visitors to offices or departments in plant; miscellaneous filing; addressing and stamping mailings; sorting and delivering incoming and outgoing mail. Responsibilities have remained the same.

4. *Do you have special training for this job?* No, but did this kind of work on my first job; would like to go to secretarial school.

5. *What do you not like about your work?* Noisy; sometimes too much to do; don't always feel like working, daydream too much; don't like the way some men look at me.

6. *What do you like best about your work?* Something to do, people are friendly, get paycheck; better than assembly line; my boss is nice to me.

7. *What is the work environment like (physical environment, atmosphere, etc.)?* Noisy; have my own desk off front lobby at entrance to room where secretarial pool, personnel, and bookkeeping offices are — all separated by partitions; people friendly.

8. *Do you have a work supervisor or boss? Is this person directly or indirectly in charge of your work? Do you work for persons other than your supervisor or boss? What kind of person is he/she?* Boss: a man, office manager; his secretary also gives me work to do. Nice man, but getting divorced; it's my fault. [Why?] Because I'm divorced and he's nice to me. He talks to me in church, sometimes buys me lunch. He notices other women; not good.

9. *How is your work organized? Do you plan what and how you do your work, or does your supervisor?* Boss or his secretary gives me work to do, e.g., filing, mailings, messages to deliver; do things when given to me. Answer telephone when it rings; answer questions; give directions when people ask; sort mail and put in boxes twice a day — 10 A.M. and 3 P.M.

10. *Do you work alone or with other people?* Work mostly alone, although talk to people on telephone and when I give directions; also when boss or secretary gives me work to do; sometimes people talk to me when they walk by my desk.

11. *What are the people like that you work with? Are you friendly with them? Do you socialize with them outside your work?* People friendly; eat lunch with secretaries in cafeteria and walk to bus with them; sometimes go out for a drink. Don't like the way some men look at me or things they say. All they're interested in is your body.

12. *Is your salary adequate? What do you do with the money that you earn?* Salary okay. Could make more if a secretary, but need training; use money for movies, bars, sometimes clothes or presents for parents, children. Try to save some to have if don't work and to help parents out.

13. *Would you like to keep this job the way it is or are there things you would like to change about it?* Job is okay for now, but will probably have to get a new job because of boss's divorce. Would like to be secretary to make more money. Wish I didn't have to work; husband's fault. He's no good.

14. *How and why did you choose this job?* Looked in newspaper. Parents and priest helped me. [Why chosen?] Because I did this work before, sort of like a secretary. Don't like assembly line, although can make more money.

Part II: Other Work Experience

1. *What other kinds of work have you done (place, job description, reasons for leaving, etc.)?*

   a. Waitress — summers, part-time during high school — quit because pregnant.

  b. Receptionist/clerk (Longshoremen's Association) — after high school, three to four years; fun, met lots of people, including husband; quit to travel and be with husband, a mistake.
  c. Assembly line (electronics firm) — after second child, to earn money; there nine months; quit to travel and be with husband; also boring, dirty.
  d. Salesgirl (dress shop) — after third child, to earn money; there two months; didn't like boss (male); low salary.
2. *Do you have work skills or special training in addition to those you have already mentioned?*
  No.

Part III: Vocational Interests and Plans
1. *What are or were your parents' occupations? Did they like their work?*
  Retired. Father worked for transport company, mother on assembly line. Didn't have much money. Parents worked hard, always wanted the best for me. Wish I hadn't disappointed them.
2. *What did you want to be as a child?*
  Movie actress or nurse.
3. *Did your parents have any influence on your job choice or career?*
  They wanted me to go to secretarial school.
4. *What other persons or events influenced your job choice or career?*
  (Laughs) Men; they're no good. I should have listened to my parents and followed teachings of the church.
5. *Which of the jobs you have had did you like the best? Why?*
  a. First job at Longshoremen's Association — fun, met lots of people; those were the good days.
  b. Current job.
6. *Which of the jobs you have had did you like the least? Why?*
  a. Assembly line — boring, dirty.
  b. Salesgirl — customers too picky, boss a "dirty old man," low salary.
7. *What three jobs or kinds of work do you feel you would be most interested in doing at this present time or in the future?*
  a. Secretary in a fancy company.
  b. Hairdresser.

   c. (Laughs.) Housewife, with a good husband — (Aside comment: Maybe I should be a whore.)

8. *What are your current work plans?*

Don't know; maybe go to secretarial school. Wish I didn't have to work.

Could go back to my job if boss wasn't getting divorced.

Part IV: Other Pertinent Information (e.g., from Employer, Family, Client)

Phone conversation with employer: Aware of MS's concern re his divorce. Feels MS is oversensitive and blames herself for others' problems. No realistic basis for MS to blame herself re his divorce. Knows MS's family through church. They're good, hard-working people. MS has had a rough life. MS overly concerned about her appearance and about making mistakes, but a conscientious, hard worker. Could take more initiative, be less timid. If MS had more secretarial skills, could give her more responsibility and a raise. Would very much like to have MS come back to work for him. (Seems concerned re MS's welfare, but no indication of inappropriate employer/employee relationship.)

Notes on Discussion with Client about Her Activity Configuration*

— Surprised, spend so much time at bars and watching TV — I really waste my life away.

— Guess I don't spend much time with my kids or help my parents out. I'm not a very good mother, should have listened to my parents. If my husband wasn't a bum, my life wouldn't be such a mess. Don't know what I'd do if my parents didn't take care of kids. I should, but I don't think I could do it, I'm too mixed up.

— Wish I had a good husband to take care of me and the kids, then maybe I would be a good mother.

— Maybe if I had some hobbies or a husband who loved me, I wouldn't be bored and waste so much time watching TV and going out.

— Wish I didn't have to work, but then I'd really be bored and that wouldn't be good.

*N.B.: Leisure and Activities of Daily Living are not included here, but they are to be investigated in the same way.

— Looks like a pretty boring life; wish it were different, but don't know what would change it except a good husband. Maybe if my husband came back to me (becomes very tearful) . . . maybe I'd be better off dead . . . . I guess I'd like things to be better, but just don't know how.

Therapist's Summary (with Interpretation)
— Use of time fairly well balanced between work, leisure, and activities of daily living pursuits; however, balance depends heavily on parents, who assume all household and child care responsibilities.
— Narrow range of social and leisure activities.
— Strong dependence on others (desire for good husband and parents).
— Little sense of choice or options; passively accepts what is available.
— Externalizes problems.
— Oriented to immediate need satisfaction.
— Concrete, unrealistic perception of relationship with husband.
— Limited insight.
— Although concerned about parents and children, has little sense of responsibility toward them; very ambivalent about child care and family activities and responsibilities.
— Low self-esteem.
— Oriented toward love and belonging needs with limited resources for mastery and esteem needs.
— Fills time more than planning or using it to meet needs in goal-oriented manner.
— Question of suicidal potential.

Appendix 3. Suggestions for Categories to be Included in Activities History*

Childhood Activities
1. Toys
2. Games
3. School subjects
4. People in activities
5. Play
6. Groups
7. Career projections
8. Chores

Adult Activities
1. Education
2. Career choices
3. Work
4. Hobbies and pastimes
5. Social activities
6. Groups
7. Recreations
8. People in activities
9. Chores

Likes and Dislikes
Ways of Spending Time
Budgeting Time
A Typical Day
Vacations
Possessions

Activities ___ chosen   ___ prescribed by others ___ just happened
Activities ___ alone   ___ with others (state who)
Activities ___ would like but _____

Activities clock: Hours per week $\left\{ \begin{array}{ll} \text{Work} & \text{Social} \\ \text{Leisure} & \text{Recreational} \\ \text{Chores} & \text{Sleep} \end{array} \right.$

*Add your own categories to those suggested here.

Each Activity:
____ Daily ____ Every other day ____ Weekly ____ Occasionally
____ Approved by group ____ Not approved by group

Read Nystrom [51] again.

Appendix 4. Worksheet for Summary of Approaches to Treatment of Dysfunction Based on a Theoretical Rationale

Theoretical approach or system of therapy (give full descriptive title):

Originator:
Followers:

Techniques advocated (step-by-step description):

Underlying rationale:

Examine:

Theory
{
Statements about the human
  condition
Descriptions of a functional
  individual
Developmental stages by which
  functional condition is
  reached
}

Therapy
{
Reasons for dysfunction
Stages that lead to
  dysfunction
Ways to reach function
  despite dysfunction
Ways to reverse dysfunction
Mechanisms by which change
  takes place
Time period in which change
  takes place
}

Occupational Therapy
Indications for clinical application (areas of dysfunction, age groups, individual patient/client considerations):

Relationship to activities frame of reference:

___ Fits in with use of therapeutic activities (how?)

___ Fits in with use of therapeutic activities with the following modifications or adjustments:

___ Does not fit in with use of therapeutic activities

Appendix 5. Protocol for Cooperative Group (Identity versus Role Confusion)

This group is characterized by shared activity, expressed in shared task goals and engagement in shared interpersonal transactions, both collaborative and competitive. The leadership remains constant (i.e., the leader is always the therapist), to represent "leader" in the larger sociocultural context — the boss, supervisor, instructor, chairperson — whose style may be authoritarian or democratic, who sets standards and exerts final decision-making power but also guides, facilitates, and negotiates. The role of each participant changes to allow for the greatest possible number of permutations in interpersonal relationships. In Erikson's terms, this group is directed to the development in the individual of a sense of identity, which is built on a sense of trust, a sense of self-control (autonomy), a sense of purpose (initiative), and a sense of competence (industry), already in some measure attained. The ethos of the group is "idealism."

Purpose of the Group
To provide a series of action situations that allow for testing a variety of roles with leader and peer role models, each representing a sampling from a different reference group. Engagement in a number of interpersonal transactions that lead to integration of ego skills, reliance on inner controls, a feeling of comfort with the self, and a coming to terms with the exigencies of the real without sacrificing the ideal are emphasized; at the same time excessive reliance on a reference group for support, overidentification with an ideal prototype, underestimation of the self, or complete rejection of social values and institutions as less than ideal are minimized. The thrust of the group is toward increasing self-confidence and self-reliance in readiness for the intimacy (in Erikson's sense) that will enable the individual to establish significant and enduring relationships with others.

139

Criteria for Admission
1. Male and female (age 16 and up)
2. Strengths:
   a. ability to communicate verbally
   b. ability to tolerate a group setting necessitating interaction with peers and with authority
   c. ability to tolerate some measure of change
   d. ability to follow instructions, verbal and written
   e. ability to concentrate, organize thinking, and reason from basic premises (basic problem-solving ability)
   f. ability to make choices
3. Problems:
   a. inability to complete a task
   b. discomfort in interpersonal relationships
   c. inability to express feelings openly and directly
   d. Perception of self as incompetent, unlikable, unworthy, or physically unappealing
   e. Alignment with a reference group counter to the existing culture (e.g., drug culture)

Size of Group
Optimum: 10
Maximum: 15
Minimum: 8

Frequency of Meeting
Group meets daily, 2 hours formally. Also assignments given at weekends.

Mode of Operation
The leader is responsible for initiating expectations (including that of change); calls for suggestions regarding the group's task selection but ultimately determines which task is most suited to the purpose of the group; breaks down task into components and allocates duties to each group member, but may delegate this responsibility to others. There is constant and regular verbal communication during and between tasks

for interchange of feedback, renegotiation of goals, and changing of participant roles. As a role model the leader acts and interacts as supervisor, mentor, guide, instructor, evaluator, and mediator, intervening to facilitate engagement on the part of the members and to elicit appropriate affective and cognitive responses. Members receive recognition for competence and achievement, and roles may change from coworker or competitor to supervisor, section leader, guide, resource person, or co-leader. Guest leaders representing role models who have successfully adapted to their sociocultural environment may be introduced periodically.

The tasks are selected to provide a series of experiences with peers and leaders that enable the individual to integrate his* skills as he tests himself in relation to others; to obtain a repertoire of coping mechanisms as he learns from others who have adapted successfully; and to receive support and validation for his strivings for an individual style that is compatible with his sociocultural milieu. It is when he is able to accept that compromise is an adaptive tool for reconciling reality with idealism, feelings with facts, practicality with altruism, and self with society that he is ready for the next step — the establishment of enduring and deep relationships without loss of individuality.

Tasks

Tasks are based on those activities that define adaptive group behavior in a particular sociocultural context, in this case:

1. Group arts and crafts activities: end product often for an altruistic goal, e.g., sale of articles for patient emergency fund, but also may be for personal gratification
2. Group daily living: care of work areas, lounge, library, units; shared responsibility by formation of committees
3. "Real" work situation: patient commissary, newsletter, boutiques, furniture restoration, greenhouse
4. Social outings

---

*The gender pronoun is used here only to simplify the discussion, which applies to group participants regardless of sex.

5. Leisure activities: dancing, photography, sports
6. Body movement, dance therapy: improvement of body image
7. "Now" involvement groups: ecology, health food preparation
8. Skills, e.g., hobbies, dressmaking, typing, classes, and educational groups
9. Beauty and deportment classes
10. Community exploration projects: cleaning up open areas, investigating local restaurants and shopping facilities, volunteer work in community agencies (Ys, gyms, etc.)

References and Suggested Readings

References

1. Arnheim, R. *Toward a Psychology of Art.* Berkeley: University of California Press, 1967.
2. Aschenbrenner, J. *Lifelines: Black Families in Chicago.* New York: Holt, Rinehart & Winston, 1955 (paperback, 1975).
3. Ayres, A. J. *The Development of Sensory Integrative Theory and Practice.* Dubuque, Iowa: Kendall/Hunt Publishing Co., 1974.
4. Ayres, A. J. Ontogenetic Principles in the Development of Arm and Hand Function. In *The Development of Sensory Integrative Theory and Practice.* Dubuque, Iowa: Kendall/Hunt Publishing Co., 1974.
5. Berne, E. *Games People Play: The Psychology of Human Relationships.* New York: Ballantine (paperback), 1976.
6. Blythe, R. *Akenfield: Portrait of an English Village.* New York: Dell (paperback), 1973.
7. Bobath, K., and Bobath, B. The neurodevelopmental treatment of cerebral palsy. *Phys. Ther.* 47:1039, 1967.
8. Bruner, J. *Towards a Theory of Instruction.* Cambridge, Mass.: The Belknap Press of Harvard University Press, 1966.
9. Bruner, J. The Will to Learn. In *Towards a Theory of Instruction.* Cambridge, Mass.: The Belknap Press of Harvard University Press, 1966. Chapter 6, pp. 113-128.
10. Brunnstrom, S. Motor behavior of adult hemiplegic patients. *Am. J. Occup. Ther.* 15:6, 1961.
11. Brunnstrom, S. *Movement Therapy in Hemiplegia.* New York: Harper & Row, 1970.
12. Buck, R. E., and Provancher, M. A. Magazine picture collages as an evaluation technique. *Am. J. Occup. Ther.* 26:1, 1972.
13. Chapin, F. S., Jr. *Human Activity Patterns in the City.* New York: Wiley, 1974.
14. Cratty, B. J. *Movement Behavior and Motor Learning* (3rd ed.). Philadelphia: Lea & Febiger, 1973.
15. Curle, A. A theoretical approach to action research. *Hum. Relations* 2:271, 1949.
16. Currie, C. Evaluating function of mentally retarded children

through the use of toys and play activities. *Am. J. Occup. Ther.* 23:35, 1969.

17. Dennis, W. *Group Values Through Children's Drawings.* New York: Wiley, 1966.

18. Diasio, K. Psychiatric occupational therapy: Search for a conceptual framework in light of psychoanalytic ego psychology and learning theory. *Am. J. Occup. Ther.* 22,5:400, 1968.

19. Erikson, E. H. *Childhood and Society* (2nd ed.). New York: Norton, 1964.

20. Erikson, E. H. Eight Ages of Man. In *Childhood and Society* (2nd ed.). New York: Norton, 1964. Chapter 7.

21. Eysenck, H. J. (Ed.). *Experiments in Behavior Therapy: Readings in Modern Methods of Treatment of Mental Disorders Derived from Learning Theory.* New York: Pergamon Press, 1964.

22. Fidler, J., and Fidler, G. *Occupational Therapy: A Communication Process in Psychiatry.* New York: Macmillan, 1963.

23. Frank, J. D., and Powdermaker, F. B. *Group Psychotherapy.* Westport, Conn.: Greenwood Press, 1973.

24. Freud, S. *A General Introduction to Psychoanalysis.* Garden City, N.Y.: Permabooks, 1954. Rev. ed.: New York: Touchstone Books (Simon & Schuster), 1969.

25. Freud, S. *Therapy and Technique.* New York: Collier Books, 1963.

26. Gesell, A. *The First 5 Years of Life.* New York: Harper, 1940.

27. Gesell, A., and Ilg, F. *The Child from 5 to 10.* New York: Harper & Row, 1977.

28. Gesell, A., and Ilg, F. *Youth: The Years from 10 to 16.* New York: Harper, 1956.

29. Glasser, W. *Reality Therapy: A New Approach to Psychiatry.* New York: Harper & Row (paperback), 1975.

30. Harlow, H. F. In Schrier, A. M., and Stollnitz, F. (Eds.), *Behavior of Non-Human Primates: Modern Research Trends,* Vol. 1 and 2. New York: Academic Press, 1965.

31. Havighurst, R. J. *Developmental Tasks and Education* (2nd ed.). London: Longmans, Green, 1952. Out of print but available in some libraries.

32. Hein, E. C. *Communication in Nursing Practice.* Boston: Little, Brown, 1973.

33. Helm, J., and Lurie, N. O. *The Dogrib Hand Game,* National Museum of Canada Bulletin No. 20, Anthropology Series 71. Ottawa: National Museum of Canada, 1966.

34. Hilgard, E. R., and Bower, G. A. *Theories of Learning* (4th ed.). New York: Appleton-Century-Crofts, 1975.

35. Holt, J. *How Children Learn.* New York: Dell (paperback), 1972.
36. Hurlock, E. B. *Child Growth and Development* (3rd ed.). New York: McGraw-Hill, 1968.
37. Hurlock, E. B. *Adolescent Development* (4th ed.). New York: McGraw-Hill, 1973.
38. Kluckhohn, C., and Leighton, D. C. *Children of the People.* Cambridge, Mass.: Harvard University Press, 1946.
39. Kluckhohn, C., and Leighton, D. C. *The Navaho* (rev. ed.). Cambridge, Mass.: Harvard University Press, 1974.
40. Kluckhohn, C., and Murray, H. A. *Personality in Nature, Society and Culture* (2nd ed.). New York: Knopf, 1961.
41. Leitenberg, H. (Ed.). *Behavior Modification: Handbook of Behavior Modification and Behavior Therapy.* Englewood Cliffs, N.J.: Prentice-Hall, 1976.
42. Lévi-Strauss, C. *Tristes Tropiques.* New York: Atheneum, 1975.
43. Liebow, E. *Tally's Corner: A Study of Negro Streetcorner Men.* Boston: Little, Brown, 1967.
44. Lifton, W. M. *Groups Facilitating Individual Growth and Social Change.* New York: Wiley, 1972.
45. Llorens, L. A. Facilitating growth and development: The promise of occupational therapy. *Am. J. Occup. Ther.* 24:93, 1967.
46. Maslow, A. *Toward a Psychology of Being* (2nd ed.). Princeton, N.J.: Van Nostrand, 1968.
47. Matsutsuyu, J. S. The interest check list. *Am. J. Occup. Ther.* 23: 323, 1969.
48. Moorehead, L. The occupational therapy history. *Am. J. Occup. Ther.* 23:329, 1969.
49. Mosey, A. C. *Three Frames of Reference for Mental Health.* Thorofare, N.J.: Charles B. Slack, 1970.
50. Mosey, A. C. The concept and use of developmental groups. *Am. J. Occup. Ther.* 24:272, 1970.
51. Nystrom, E. P. Activity patterns and leisure concepts among the elderly. *Am. J. Occup. Ther.* 28:337, 1974.
52. Opie, I., and Opie, P. *Children's Games in Street and Playground.* Oxford: Clarendon Press, 1969.
53. Piaget, J., and Inhelder, B. *The Psychology of the Child.* New York: Basic Books, 1969.
54. Phillips, E. L., and Wiener, D. N. Writing Therapy: A New Approach to Treatment and Training. In *Short-term Psychotherapy and Structured Behavior Change.* New York: McGraw-Hill, 1966.
55. Poggie, J. J., Jr., and Gersuny, C. *Fishermen of Galilee: The Human Ecology of a New England Coastal Community,* University of

Rhode Island Marine Bulletin, Series 17. Narragansett, R.I.: University of Rhode Island, 1974.

56. Rasch, P. J., and Burke, R. K. *Kinesiology and Applied Anatomy* (5th ed.). Philadelphia: Lea & Febiger, 1974.

57. Reilly, M. Occupational therapy can be one of the great ideas of twentieth century medicine. *Am. J. Occup. Ther.* 26:1, 1962.

58. Reilly, M. (Ed.). *Play as Explorative Learning.* Beverly Hills, Calif.: Russell Sage, 1974.

59. Roberts, J. M., Arth, M. J., and Bush, R. R. Games in culture. *Am. Anthro.* 61:599, 1959.

60. Rogers, C. *Client-Centered Therapy.* Boston: Houghton Mifflin, 1951.

61. Rood, M. S. Neurophysiological mechanisms utilized in the treatment of neuromuscular dysfunction. *Am. J. Occup. Ther.* 4 (1956): Part II, 220.

62. Ruesch, J. *Therapeutic Communication.* New York: Norton, 1973.

63. Sagan, C. *The Cosmic Connection.* New York: Doubleday, 1973.

64. Sager, C. J., and Kaplan, H. S. *Progress in Group and Family Therapy.* New York: Brunner/Mazel, 1972.

65. Scarry, R. *What Do People Do All Day.* New York: Random House, 1968.

66. Stieper, D. R., and Wiener, D. N. *Dimensions of Psychotherapy.* Chicago: Aldine, 1965.

67. Szalai, A. (Ed.). *The Use of Time: Daily Activities of Urban and Suburban Populations in Twelve Countries.* The Hague: Mouton, 1972.

68. Takata, N. The play history. *Am. J. Occup. Ther.* 23:314, 1969.

69. White, R. W. Motivation reconsidered: The concept of competence. In Rabkin, L. Y., and Carr, J. E. (Eds.), *Sourcebook of Abnormal Psychology.* Boston: Houghton Mifflin, 1967.

70. World Federation of Occupational Therapists. *Cultural Patterns and Their Influence on Rehabilitation,* Proceedings of Third International Congress. Philadelphia: the Federation, 1962.

71. Worth, S., and Adair, J. Navajo filmmakers. *Am. Anthro.* 72:9, 1970.

72. Zimmerman, M. Devices: Development and direction. *Am. J. Occup. Ther.,* AOTA Conference Issue, 1960.

Suggested Readings

Special Note: *American Journal of Occupational Therapy. Special AOTA 60th Anniversary 1917-1977 Commemorative Issue:* A retrospective and prospective view of occupational therapy. Vol. 31, November–December 1977.

American Journal of Physical Medicine. An Exploratory and Analytical Survey of Therapeutic Exercise, North West University Therapeutic Exercise Project. Baltimore: Williams & Wilkins, 1967.

Argyris, C. Theories of action that inhibit individual learning. *Am. Psychol.* 31:638, 1976.

Basmajian, J. V. *Muscles Alive* (3rd ed.). Baltimore: Williams & Wilkins, 1974.

Bauer, B. A. Tactile sensitivity: Development of a behavioral responses checklist. *Am. J. Occup. Ther.* 31:357, 1977.

Berlson, B., and Steiner, G. *Human Behavior: An Inventory of Scientific Findings.* New York: Harcourt, Brace & World, 1964.

Bronfenbrenner, U. Towards an experimental ecology of human development. *Am. Psychol.* 32:513, 1977.

Cermak, S. A., Stein, F., and Abelson, C. Hyperactive children and an activity group model. *Am. J. Occup. Ther.* 27:311, 1973.

Damon, A., Stroudt, H., and McFarland, R. *The Human Body in Equipment Design.* Cambridge, Mass.: Harvard University Press, 1966.

Estes, W. K. The cognitive side of probability learning. *Psychiatr. Rev.* 83:37, 1976.

Fabun, D. *The Dynamics of Change.* Englewood Cliffs, N.J.: Prentice-Hall, 1968.

Fogel, V., and Rosillo, R. Correlation of psychological variables and progress in physical rehabilitation. *Dis. Nerv. Syst.* 30:593, 1969.

Ford, D., and Urban, H. *Systems of Psychotherapy: A Comparative Study.* New York: Wiley, 1963.

Freud, S. *Psychopathology of Everyday Life.* New York: Norton, 1971.

Freud, S. *Civilization and Its Discontents.* New York: Norton, 1962.

Hasselkus, B., and Safrit, M. J. Measurement in occupational therapy. *Am. J. Occup. Ther.* 30:429, 1976.

Heine, D. B. Daily living group: Focus on transition from hospital to community. *Am. J. Occup. Ther.* 29:628, 1975.

Heron, A. *Why Men Work.* Stanford, Calif.: Stanford University Press, 1948. Out of print but available in some libraries.

Isaac, S., and Michael, W. B. *Handbook in Research and Evaluation.* San Diego, Calif.: Edits, 1977.

Jones, M. *The Therapeutic Community.* New York: Basic Books, 1953.

Jones, M. *Beyond the Therapeutic Community.* New Haven, Conn.: Yale University Press, 1968.

Jung, C. *Man and His Symbols.* New York: Doubleday, 1969.

Kottak, C. P. *Cultural Anthropology.* New York: Random House, 1975. See especially Chapter 12, Culture and Personality, and Chapter 13, The Anthropology of Complex Societies; also, Sources and Suggested Readings.

Kroeber, A. L. *Anthropology: Culture Patterns and Processes.* New York: Harbinger (Harcourt, Brace & World), 1963.

Lazarus, A. A. Has behavior therapy outlived its usefulness? *Am. Psychol.* 32:550, 1977.

Lewko, J. H. Current practices in evaluating motor behavior of disabled children. *Am. J. Occup. Ther.* 30:413, 1976.

Llorens, L. A. Activity analysis for cognitive-perceptual-motor dysfunction. *Am. J. Occup. Ther.* 27:453, 1973.

Luria, A. R. *Higher Cortical Functions in Man.* New York: Basic Books, 1973.

Maluccio, A. N. Action as a tool in casework practice. *Soc. Casework,* p. 30, 1974.

Marmo, N. A. Discovering the lifestyle of the physically disabled. *Am. J. Occup. Ther.* 29:475, 1975.

Meacham, R., and Lindemann, J. E. A summer program for underachieving adolescents. *Am. J. Occup. Ther.* 29:280, 1975.

Mechanic, D., Lewis, C., and Fein, R. *A Right to Health.* New York: Wiley, 1976.

Menks, F., Sittler, S., Weaver, D., and Yanow, R. A psychogeriatric group in a rural community. *Am. J. Occup. Ther.* 31:376, 1977.

Michaels, E. Associated movements and motor learning. *Phys. Ther.* 50:24, 1970.

Morrow, W. R. *Behavior Therapy Bibliography 1950-1969.* Columbia, Miss.: University of Mississippi Press, 1971.

Mumford, M. S. A comparison of interpersonal skills in verbal and activity groups. *Am. J. Occup. Ther.* 28:281, 1974.

Oeri, G. *Man and His Images: A Way of Seeing.* New York: Viking, 1968.

Pieper, J. *Leisure, the Basis of Culture.* New York: New American Library, 1964.

Quest, I., and Cordery, J. A functional ulnar deviation cuff for the rheumatoid deformity. *Am. J. Occup. Ther.* 25:32, 1971.

Richards, M. *Centering in Pottery, Poetry, and the Person.* Middletown, Conn.: Wesleyan University Press, 1964.

Schwartzman, H. B. The anthropological study of children's play. *Annu. Rev. Anthro.* 5:289, 1976.

Shannon, P. Work-play theory. *Am. J. Occup. Ther.* 26:169, 1972.

UNESCO. *The Arts and Man: A World View of the Role and Functions of the Arts in Society.* Englewood Cliffs, N.J.: Prentice-Hall, 1969. Out of print but available in some libraries.

Vygotsky, L. S. *Thought and Language.* Cambridge, Mass.: MIT Press, 1962.

White, R. W. The urge towards competence. *Am. J. Occup. Ther.* 25: 271, 1971.

World Federation of Occupational Therapists. *Occupational Therapy Today – Tomorrow.* Proceedings, 5th International Congress. Zurich: the Federation, 1970.

Yerxa, E. Authentic occupational therapy. *Am. J. Occup. Ther.* 21:1, 1967.

Index

Index